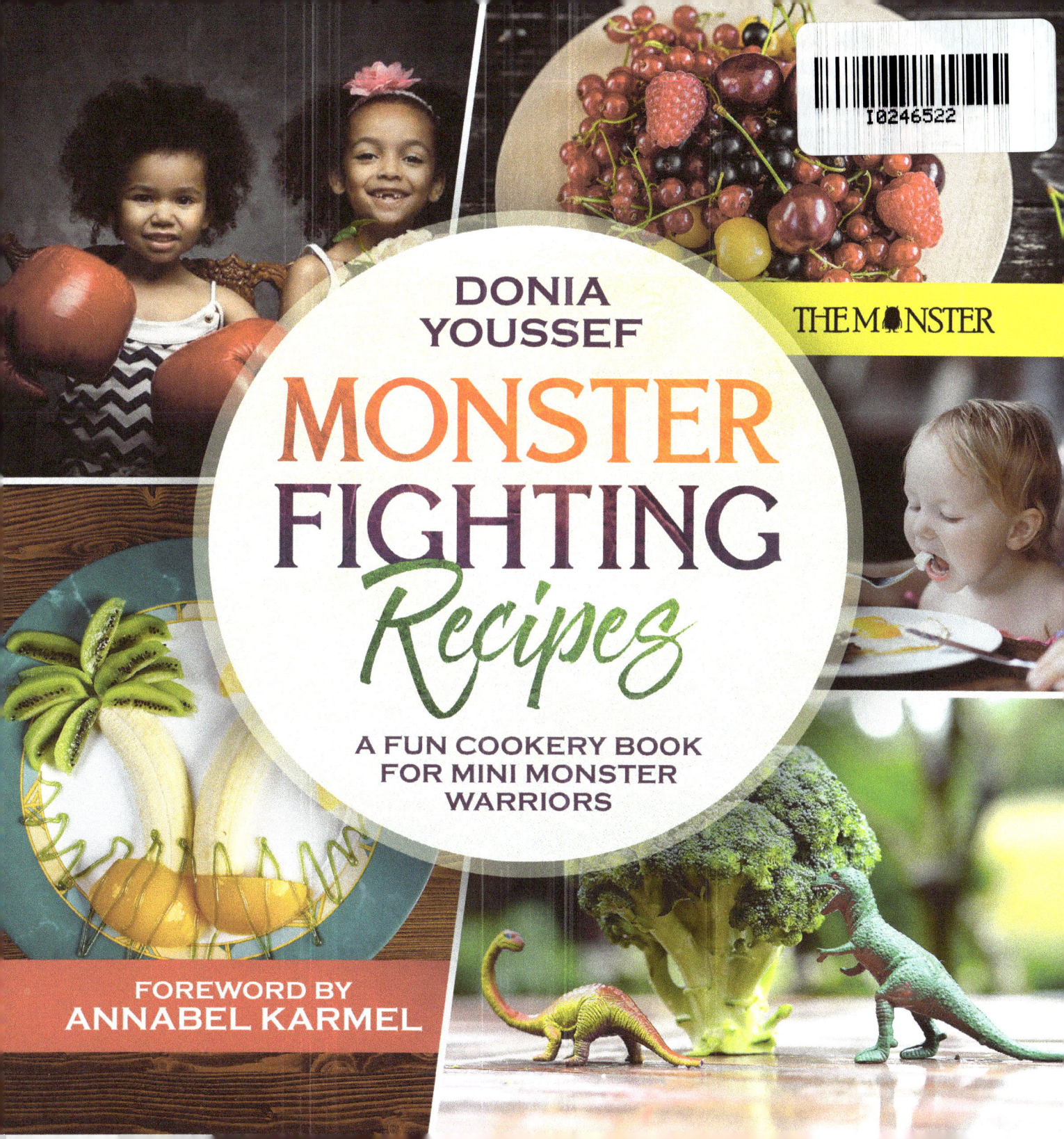

Copyright© 2019 Tiny Angel Press LTD.

All rights reserved. No part of this book may be reproduced, stored in a retrieval system or transmitted in any form or by any means, electronic, electrostatic, magnetic tape, mechanical, photocopying, recording or otherwise, without the prior permission in writing of the publisher.

ISBN: 978-1-9162194-2-7

THE MONSTER SERIES
Published by Tiny Angel Press LTD.
Layout Design: Nonon Tech & Design

Disclaimers

The materials contained in this book are provided for general information purposes only and do not constitute legal or other professional advice on any subject matter. Monster Repelling Recipes Book does not accept any responsibility for any loss which may arise from reliance on information contained in this book.

This book and its contents are provided 'AS IS' without warranty of any kind, either express or implied, including, but not limited to, the implied warranties of merchantability, fitness for a particular purpose, or non-infringement.

Acknowledgement

Putting a book of this nature together has been a goal of mine for some time. Seeing it take shape has been an emotional experience for me as it was something I decided I wanted to create whilst I was in the midst of my own cancer journey. I can remember the specific moment it came to me whilst sitting in my hospital chair, wired up to chemotherapy and trying to get enthusiastic about food, any food to keep my energy up!

What has made me even more emotional is the outpouring of generosity and enthusiasm from all the chefs and cooks who have kindly donated recipes for the book! Annabel Karmel, Jen Hansard, Phillipa Barlow, Pete Evans, Rishim Sachdeva, Sarah Almond Bushell and the amazing team at MacMillan Cancer Support, it has been a joy collaborating with you all. Thank you so very much for embracing my project and adding your exceptional culinary and nutritional expertise and advice to make it such a success. I know there are going to be many, many families, worldwide who, at such a horrendous time in their lives, are going to now benefit from your healthy, delicious, not to mention, fun recipes!

A big thank you to Louise Wyatt for coming up with the book title!

A huge thank you to the truly incredible Royal Marsden Hospital for all their help and support both to me personally and with all my cancer awareness campaigns.

And finally, I would like to personally say thank you to Tamara, for selflessly contributing many mouth watering recipes written specifically for this book. The ingredients have been selected for their powerful inner healing qualities, and each recipe includes the nutritional benefits to help re-educate us on the importance of nourishment and self-care.

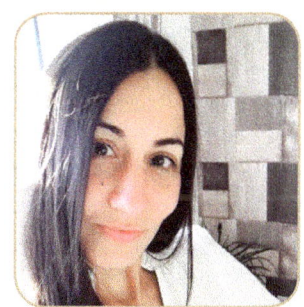

Tamara is a renowned Total Wellness Therapist, with more than 15 years of experience in Health and Wellbeing.

She is the founder of Breathe360, a revolutionary, Holistic Health Service that offers a comprehensive approach for you and your family's total health and wellbeing.

Through years of research, study and self-healing, Breathe360 offers tool-kits that help you take back your health and deliver long term positive results.

Involved in a serious road traffic accident at the age of 19, Tamara was left to survive on heavy medication and metalwork in her spine. In 2004, she requested all metalwork to be removed, and changed her life path, stopping all forms of medication, and through her own personal Journey, has ultimately created Breathe360.

Tamara has used many tried and tested methods, experienced many unwanted symptoms, and managed to restore her energy for Life. Her focus is on getting to the root of your health using scientific techniques and applying them holistically to help re-energise your system by releasing energy blocks, and optimise cell communication. The building blocks, that she believes is required for living a healthy and happy life. Tamara empowers you to heal from the inside out, adopt a healthy lifestyle, and feel better fast using self-help toolkits.

The shop and wellness centre is nestled in Lyndhurst, Hampshire offering treatments, with natural products and supplements to further support your health journey and total wellbeing. Retreats are hosted at their dedicated House in Oxfordshire.

Breathe360 brings together a personal journey of knowledge and lifestyle, creating a wonderful ambience where you are welcomed by Tamara and her Team.

The intent is to help prevent others from going through the challenges that Tamara faced for many years. Breathe360 is not just a brand it is a lifestyle.

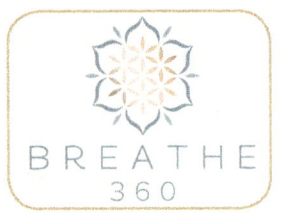

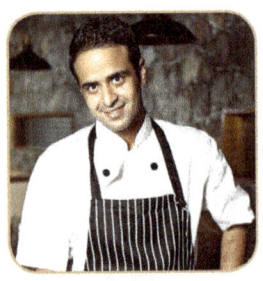

Rishim Sachdeva: Love of fresh and local ingredients. Leaning towards techniques like fermenting and preserving, marrying classic with modern and create varied flavours.

What started as a chance encounter with a bitter but delicious apricot kernel at age 6, some cooking lessons from his mum, has ended up taking Chef Rishim Sachdeva to the kitchens of Michelin star restaurants. Marco Pierre White's The Oakroom at the mere age of 18 and Heston Blumenthal's legendary Fat Duck. Having mastered the classic French cooking techniques, Chef Rishim then moved to a more molecular, then eventually more nordic style of cooking.

A lover of seasonal, fresh, local ingredients, Chef Rishim leans towards classic techniques like fermenting and preserving, processes that enable one to extract flavours and textures that last through the year. He's a fan of cooking with lesser ingredients rather than adding more to improve the flavour of the dish.

Currently spearheading Mumbai's iconic Olive Bar & Kitchen, he's brought his style of cooking on to the menu with dishes like Apple and Pork, Cauliflower and Date, Red Velvet Fried Chicken and many more. Ask him what his favourite creation is up until now and he says, 'It changes every week!'.

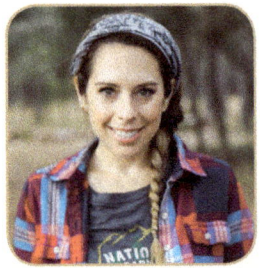

Jen Hansard, the personality of Simple Green Smoothies, is on a fresh path to health and happiness- deprivation not included. Her 'healthy obsession' with green smoothies has taken her into classrooms to do green smoothie demos, lead entrepreneur workshops, speak on stage, and has been featured on The Doctors to spread the plant-powered love far and wide. Through the power of green smoothies, she's seen the amazing health benefits first-hand – including more energy, which has been the catalyst to healthy living for Jen and her family.

Her wildly popular website, SimpleGreenSmoothies.com, has changed the lives of over 1 million people and is the #1 green smoothie online resource. The Simple Green Smoothies' lifestyle doesn't involve counting calories or eliminating an entire food group. Instead, it encourages you to make one simple change: drink one green smoothie a day. Jen lives in Brooksville, Florida with her husband, two lil' rawkstars Jackson and Clare... and their pet chickens, ducks and dog.

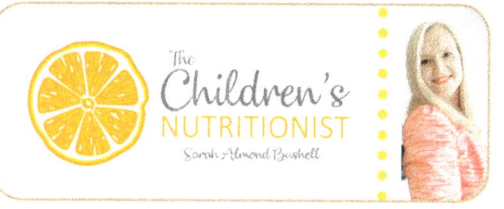

Sarah Almond Bushell

The Children's Nutritionist

An award winning Registered Dietitian, Children's Nutritionist & Baby Weaning Expert. She helps families nourish their babies and children through food, recipes, nutrition and feeding habits.

www.childrensnutrition.co.uk

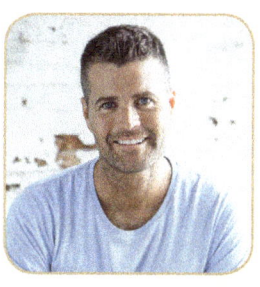

Pete Evans is an internationally renowned and household chef, restaurateur, author and television presenter. His passion for food and a healthy lifestyle inspires individuals and families around the world.

A love of food saw Pete begin his career as chef and restaurateur at the age of 19, opening numerous award-winning restaurants nationally as well as cooking in some of the finest restaurants globally

As an in-demand keynote speaker on healthy eating, wellness and sustainability, he loves to share his knowledge and educate all generations, from parents and children to corporate audiences.

www.peteevans.com

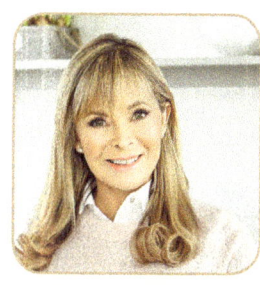

Annabel Karmel: With a career spanning over 25 years, London born mother of three, Annabel Karmel, has pioneered the way families all over the world feed their babies and children.

Credited with starting a food revolution with her trusty recipes and methods, she has become the UKs No.1 children's cookery author, best-selling international author, and the mother of all feeding experts with 45 cookbooks...and counting.

www.annabelkarmel.com

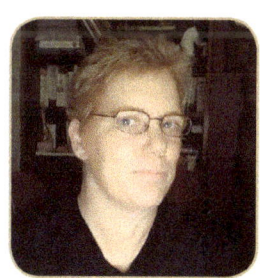

Phillipa Barlow is a mother of three children and has spent most of her life travelling. She became a Cordon Bleu Chef and through this, she went into Hospitality and Property Estate Management within the High End and VIP market. In 2017 she was diagnosed with Breast Cancer and while having treatment, she took up Art and Sculpture. After completing treatment, she was offered a Place at University, to study Contemporary Fine art. Through this course, she is able to express herself and potentially help others work through their issues in life, utilising Art as Therapy..

www.pipclaireart.co.uk

MACMILLAN CANCER SUPPORT

Macmillan Cancer Support is registered as a charity with the Charity Commission (registered charity number 261017) and as a company limited by guarantee with the Registrar of Companies (registered company number 2400969).

www.macmillan.org.uk

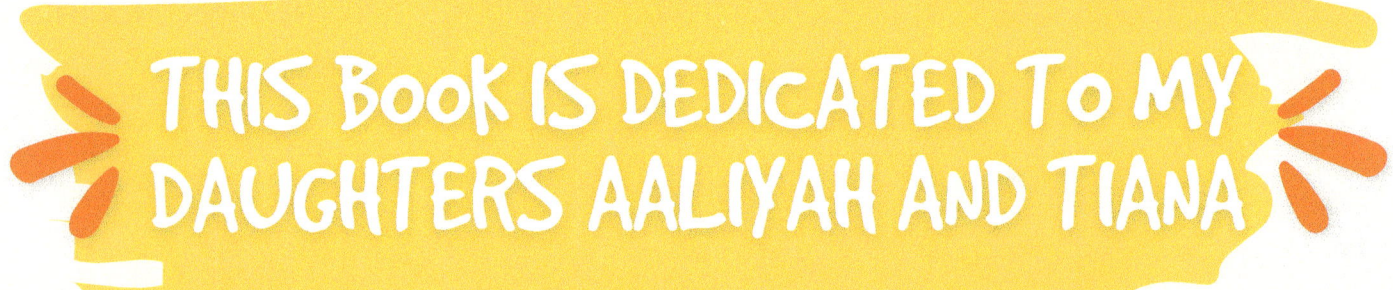
THIS BOOK IS DEDICATED TO MY DAUGHTERS AALIYAH AND TIANA

Table of contents

Foreword 1
Introduction 3

BREAKFAST/SNACKS

Reduced Sugar Carrot, Clementine, Poppy Seed and Parsnip Muffins 10
Banana, Honey and Hazelnut Smoothie 12
Fruit Smoothie 14
Macmillan Coco Hahona 16
Lemon Seeded Muffins 18
Choc, Vanilla & Cinnamon Smoothie 20
Celery Juice 22
Toasted Cinnamon and Vanilla Nuts 24
Pecan and Hazelnut Bread 26
Beginner's Luck 28
Carrot, Apple and Sultana Muffins 30
Butternut Squash, Leek and Parmesan Risotto 32
Vegetable Leather 34

LIGHT LUNCH

Lil' Adventurer Cauliflower Smoothie Bowl 38
Caribbean-Style Tuna Spread 40
Smoked Fish Chowder 42
Sardine bruschetta 44
Minty Summer Rice Salad 46
Parsnip and Coconut Soup 48
Rainbow Oven Omelette 50
Sweet Potato Wedges with Sour Cream and Chive Dip 52
Upside Down Mini Pizza 54
Bone Broth 56
Potassium Broth 58
Creamy Vegetable Soup 60
Oven Baked Chicken Nuggets 62
Baked Potato Mice 64
Chicken with Tomatoes and Orzo 66
Steak and Egg on Pumpkin 'Toast' 68

DINNER/MAIN MEAL

Vegan Black Bean and Lentil Chili with nacho chips	72
Lemon and Garlic Chicken	74
Pan-Fried Snapper with Broccomole	76
Sweet Potato Crab Cakes	78
Chicken and white bean salad	80
Cod Viennoise	82
Salmon curry	84
One-pot Fish with Black Olives and Tomatoes	86
Tuna and Vegetable Spaghetti	88
Spring onion, garlic and prawn risotto	90
Chicken Curry	92
Quick Shepherd's Pie	94
Speedy Moroccan Meatballs	96
Butternut Squash, Raisin and Apricot Muffins	98
Spring vegetable casserole	100
Mixed Bean Mexican Chilli	102
Fish Pie	104
Stuffed Pepper Smiley Faces	106
Mummy Favourite Fish Pie	108
Hidden Vegetable Spaghetti Bolognese	110
Tuna Pasta Bake	112
ONE DISH CHICKEN AND RICE BAKE	113
Butternut squash lasagne	114

DESSERTS/PUDDINGS

Salted Sweet Potato Caramel and Chocolate Tart	116
Summer Pudding	118
Greek Honey Cheesecake with Apricot Compote	120
Brown Sugar Plums with Sour Cream	122
Microwave Banana Pudding	124
Coconut and Cardamom Rice Pudding	126
Amaretti Stuffed Peaches	128
Beet Cupcakes	130
Raw Honey Cookie Bites	132
Avocado Icecream	134
Raspberry Mousse	136
Lemon Mint and Ginger Lollies	138

ACCOMPANIMENTS

Homemade Vegan Butter	142
South American Dressing	144

Foreword

BY ANNABEL KARMEL,
THE UK'S NO. 1 CHILDREN'S COOKERY AUTHOR & LEADING FOOD EXPERT

I first met Donia on a photo shoot we were both involved in which was all around meal ideas for children. We soon got chatting and I was interested to hear about Donia's personal cancer journey and her incredible 'Monster' book series which she developed to help raise awareness of the illness. The idea behind Donia's recipe book, 'Monster Repelling Recipes' is fantastic - it provides delicious and highly nutritious meals for children who have been given a cancer diagnosis. I have spent my whole career over the past 27 years inventing tasty, nutritiously balanced meals for babies, children and families and finding ways to encourage even the most disinterested child to eat well!

Never is food more important than when a child receives a diagnosis of a chronic illness such as cancer, and their immune system takes a severe battering as a result. Along with a depleted immune system, cancer treatment presents other issues that can make eating the last thing a child wants to do. These symptoms can include painful mouth ulcers, a dry and horrid metallic taste in the mouth and also taste buds can often stop functioning altogether, making the experience of eating food not the joyous occasion it should be and instead extremely bland and uninteresting. Even chewing can become a laborious task. However, getting nutrition through food is crucial, particularly when fighting a serious illness, when you need to keep your immune system as strong as possible and energy levels topped up to the max. As parents will know, it is not always easy to get a sick child to eat. During cancer treatment, it's often crucial that the patient keeps their calorie count up to enable them to be strong enough for treatment. Therefore, eating a healthy, nutritious diet packed with those critical nutrients is paramount. Donia's book provides recipes which are high in flavour to endeavour to keep the recipes as tasty as possible, even when those pesky taste buds are rebelling and falling short! Each recipe is also quick and simple to cook and selected to be as palatable as possible, even when energy is low and chewing might be difficult. I love the concept behind Donia's latest campaign, bringing together recipes from chefs all around the world for children affected by cancer. Not only does it help to raise awareness of the illness but it supports families going through a very difficult time and I can't recommend it enough.

Introduction

The word cancer is enough to make most people feel uneasy due to how serious this kind of diagnosis can be for a person. With that said, this becomes an even scarier problem when children are the ones affected. It is hard to believe that over 15 thousand parents per year are going to have to face a cancer diagnosis with a child.

There are more than 40 cases of childhood cancer every day, and this is a very alarming number without a doubt. Cancer a disease that knows no boundaries related to ethnicity or household economy – it can strike anyone, at any time.

One of the many concerns is that there are many types of cancer that children can suffer from, and this is often going to lead to several health issues when treating the condition. This increases the chances of mouth ulcers, weight loss, neutropenia and many other health problems that can make the recovery process much harder.

This is the reason why this book was created and the reason why I feel so passionate about the material it contains. Being someone who understands the ordeals of dealing with cancer, I went on a quest to help parents who have a child with cancer and are struggling to give their child comfort while they battle the disease.

There is very hard evidence of the importance that a healthy diet has when dealing with a disease like cancer. Being aware of this made me feel extremely committed to the process of coming up with the best possible recipes. I knew this was essential in order to help children with optimal nutrition. This way they can enjoy wholesome foods without feeling like they are eating something they won't enjoy.

This book is going to take you on a journey of optimal recipes that are going to boost your child's immune system and help them deal with cancer the right way, the natural way. This is in no way some kind of holistic replacement for cancer treatment - this is about reinforcement for the body to keep it as healthy as possible.

Nutrition has always been the key factor that allows people to live healthy and happy lives. We have all heard of the rare cases when people exercised and always consumed healthy foods, but they still had to deal with cancer and the condition was too hard to handle. The rarity of those cases is often blurred further by the lack of information on the habits that these people had their entire lives.

It is a fact that a healthy diet can be extremely helpful for people who are dealing with any kind of disease and cancer is no different. These recipes are meant to give you a powerful natural option that is going to help nourish your child to allow their bodies to handle the recovery process and the battle with cancer effectively.

I hope you and your child can get some peace of mind by knowing that this book was made for you. It was made to provide an extra light that guides you further in the path of recovery.

MORE INFORMATION TO USE AT BEGINNING OF BOOK

Eating well can help kids with cancer feel better and cope with the side effects of cancer or its treatments.

To keep up their strength and deal with side effects, kids should stay hydrated, take only doctor-recommended supplements, and eat as well as possible, even though that sometimes can be hard. For some kids undergoing treatment, that might mean getting enough to eat; for others, it could mean making sure not to eat too much.

STAYING HYDRATED

Kids being treated for cancer often lose a lot of water from vomiting, diarrhoea, or by just not drinking enough. This can lead to dehydration. To avoid it, make sure your child gets plenty of fluids. Tap, filtered, or bottled water is best, but your child can also get necessary fluids from other sources, like juices (100% juice is best) and soups.

Water helps with nearly every body function — from digestion and metabolizing fat, to flushing toxins from the body and maintaining body temperature. Getting enough fluids also helps prevent constipation, a condition that can make a child even less inclined to eat.

EATING RIGHT

Every kid with cancer has specific nutritional needs, so it's important to talk to a nutritionist about what would be best for your child. In general, kids with cancer have an increased need for protein, carbohydrates, and healthy fats.

Protein helps the body grow, repair tissues, build blood cells and replenish the immune system. Getting enough protein can help your child heal faster from the side effects of radiation and chemotherapy, while also helping to prevent infections. Foods like cheese, eggs, milk, yoghurt, lean meats, poultry, fish, beans, peanut butter, nuts, lentils, and soy are all good sources of protein.

Carbohydrates are the body's fuel, providing energy for cells and helping to maintain organ function. Good sources of carbs include breads, pasta, potatoes, rice, cereals, fruits, corn, and beans. Whole-grain bread and pasta are usually best because they add fibre, which helps kids feel fuller longer and prevents constipation, a common side effect of cancer treatment.

Fats help the body store energy, insulate body tissues, and carry certain vitamins throughout the bloodstream. Fats also are dense in calories, which is important to a child who might be losing weight during treatment. Not all fats are created equal, though.

Unsaturated fats that are found in fish, nuts, olive oil, and vegetables like avocados are much healthier than saturated fats and trans fats that are found in red meats and greasy, fried foods.

Dietary supplements usually aren't recommended, as they can interfere with some cancer treatments. Don't give your child any supplement unless your health care provider recommends it. It's best for kids to get their nutrients through food.

HELPING YOUR CHILD EAT MORE

When kids aren't feeling their best, it can be difficult to get them to eat. Try these tips to help your child:

- Offer smaller, more frequent meals. Also serve meals on a smaller plate, since a large plate of food can seem like too much to someone with a decreased appetite.
- Always have food on hand. Whether it's a breakfast bar, a liquid nutrition drink or shake, crackers, or fruit, keep snacks handy in case your child suddenly gets hungry.
- Try blander foods. If your child seems sensitive to strong smells or tastes, stick to plain meals like breads, pastas, rice, and broth-type soups.
- Experiment with food temperatures. Many kids undergoing treatment prefer foods that are served at room temperature rather than very hot or too cold.
- Avoid acidic foods. If mouth sores are a problem, stay away from acidic foods like orange juice, lemonade, and tomatoes.
- Make foods easier to swallow. If swallowing is difficult, try pureed foods, soups, shakes, or smoothies. A straw may help them go down easier.
- Don't offer liquids with meals. Serve drinks in between meals, instead of with meals. This way, your child won't fill up on fluids and will have an appetite to eat. (But if your child has mouth sores or dry mouth, offering fluids with meals actually helps the food go down.)
- Make up for lost calories. Your child might not want to eat very much when receiving chemotherapy. So in between treatments, make up for the decreased intake with things like high-calorie bars and milkshakes. Ask your child's doctor for recommendations.

HELPING YOUR CHILD EAT LESS (OR BETTER!)

Many kids undergoing cancer treatment tend to eat less and lose weight because their appetites are affected.

But some kids have increased appetites, especially if they're on steroid medicines that can make them hungrier. This can lead to fluid retention and weight gain. These problems will go away after treatment ends. But in the meantime, it's important for kids to maintain a healthy weight.

THESE TIPS CAN HELP:

> - Set a mealtime schedule. Serve three moderate-sized meals a day, plus two or three snacks, and make sure your child sticks to that schedule. Encourage your child to wait for at least 20 minutes after eating something before asking for more. (In general, it takes kids this long to realize they're full.)
> - Limit salt intake. Help prevent fluid build-up by limiting the amount of salt in your child's diet. Avoid fast foods, processed foods, frozen meals, and snacks like chips and pretzels. Use spices other than salt to season foods made at home.
> - Serve fruits and veggies first. Offer fruits and vegetables at the beginning of the meal, followed by whole-grain products (like bread and pasta). Foods like these that are high in fibre keep kids feeling fuller longer.
> - Provide healthy snacks. Keep only healthy foods in the house for snacking, and bring healthy snacks with you when you go out. Limit your child's intake of soda and sweets, which are both loaded with empty calories.
> - Stay active. Help keep your child's mind off of eating — try alternative activities, such as sports, games, reading, or hobbies. To help burn excess calories, your child should try to stay active and get plenty of exercise if he or she feels up to it.
> - Keep food out of sign and out of mind. Limit food-related TV shows and keep food in a cabinet, not out on the counter.
> - Limit liquids with calories. Juices, sodas, and sports drinks have extra calories and very little nutrition. And they don't satisfy hunger.

When the steroid or other treatment ends, your child's appetite should return to normal and may even decrease for a short time. This is normal and not typically a cause for alarm. Your child's doctor will probably be expecting the weight loss associated with this and will keep a close eye on it.

EATING TO REDUCE SIDE EFFECTS

Cancer and its treatments can cause several side effects, including nausea, vomiting, dry mouth, mouth sores, constipation, and diarrhoea. They also can:

> heighten sensitivity to food smells or temperatures

> make swallowing difficult

> cause changes in taste that might make kids not like foods they once enjoyed

Fortunately, once treatment ends, these problems go away.

In the meantime, help with nausea and vomiting by making sure your child takes all medicines correctly and eats the right things. Offer bland foods, especially on days when your child has treatment. Avoid salty, sweet, fatty, and fried foods. Food smells also can play a part in nausea. Consider offering foods with little or no smell, and don't cook hot foods around your child.

To help control diarrhoea, give your child foods like white bread, bananas, white rice, and applesauce that are easy to digest. Avoid dairy products; greasy, spicy, or fried foods; high-fibre foods; raw fruits and vegetables; and foods like cabbage and broccoli that can cause gas. Kids with diarrhoea should drink more than usual to replace lost fluids.

To help control constipation, offer your child high-fibre foods, such as fruits, vegetables, nuts, and whole-grain breads and cereals. In addition to water, give your child fruit and vegetable juices (such as prune juice), and warm liquids like tea.

A change in food preferences might seem like an insignificant problem, but if it causes your child to lose interest in eating, it won't be. You'll need to manage this for as long as it lasts, which can be weeks or even years:

> Help your child to practice good oral hygiene by brushing teeth regularly and rinsing out the mouth often — this can help decrease mouth sores and make food taste better.

> If your child is sensitive to the taste of metal, try using plastic forks and spoons instead.

> Encourage your child to try new foods. Those with strong flavors can often mask the taste changes in your child's mouth.

> Keep a wide variety of foods handy to help meet your child's changing tastes.

SAFE FOOD HANDLING AND PREP

Kids with cancer are at high risk for infection, so it's very important to know how to handle and prepare food safely. This means washing your hands well before handling food or after touching things like raw meat and poultry.

It also means things like keeping hot foods hot and cold foods cold. Prepared food should never be allowed to sit at room temperature for more than an hour, and leftovers should be eaten within a few days.

Raw fruits and veggies should always be washed well before they're eaten. This includes melons or any other thick-skinned fruit you might cut with a knife. Cooked foods should be cooked well before they're served.

ENCOURAGING GOOD EATING HABITS

When kids have trouble eating enough, it can be easy to give in and let them eat anything, healthy or not, just so they're getting some calories. But it's important to encourage healthy eating habits.

Eating nutritious foods will help make your child less likely to binge on sweets or fried foods. And remember, some day the treatment will end, and your child's appetite will go back to normal. When it does, the good eating habits built now will help your child choose healthy options.

It can be tricky to keep your child focused on nutrition during treatment, but it's important to try. Kids who eat well and stay hydrated are better able to tolerate and stay on schedule for treatments, steer clear of infections, keep a healthy weight, and stay strong enough to enjoy favourite activities — all of which increase their chances for the best possible outcome.

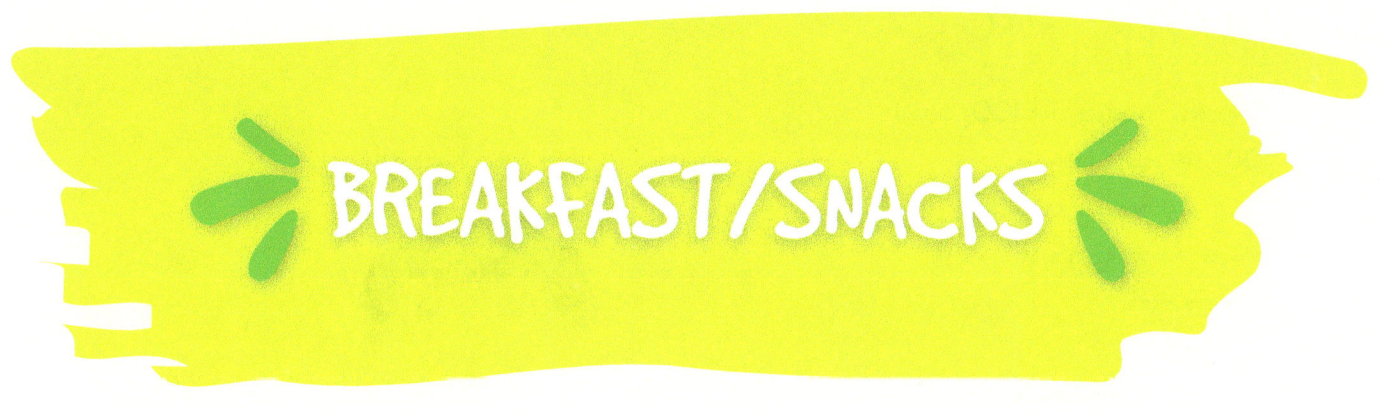

Reduced Sugar Carrot, Clementine, Poppy Seed and Parsnip Muffins

MAKES: 12 MUFFINS | PREP: 10 MINS | COOKING TIME: 25 MINS

Ingredients:

- 35g Stevia sweetener (or 100g sugar)
- 100g self raising flour
- 100g wholemeal self raising flour
- 1/4 tsp bicarbonate of soda
- 1 tsp cinnamon
- 1 tsp ginger
- 1 large parsnip peeled and grated
- 1 small carrot, peeled and grated
- Zest and juice of 2 clementine's
- 1 tbsp poppy seeds
- 50g natural yoghurt
- 75ml rapeseed oil
- 2 eggs, beaten

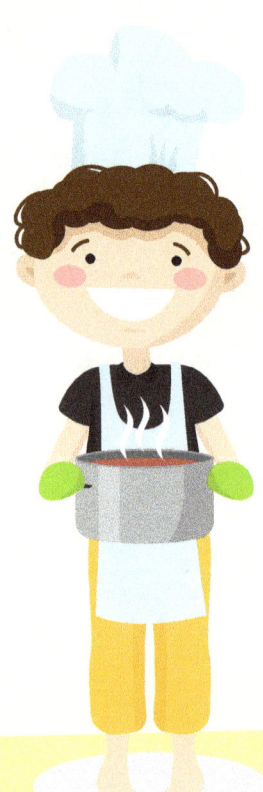

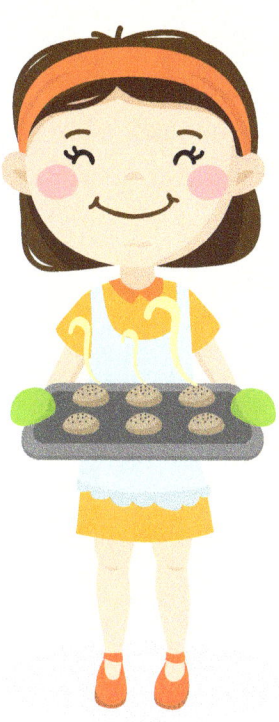

Method:

1. Prepare the carrot and parsnip as described.
2. Preheat oven to 180 degrees C.
3. Line a 12 hole muffin tray with paper cases.
4. Add the oil, stevia/sugar, yoghurt, clementine juice & zest and eggs to a bowl and mix together.
5. Stir in the grated parsnip, carrot and poppy seeds.
6. In a clean bowl combine the flours, bicarb and spices.
7. Add the wet mixture to the dry mixture and stir to combine.
8. Fill muffin cases equally. (I use an ice cream scoop) & bake for 25mins or until golden.

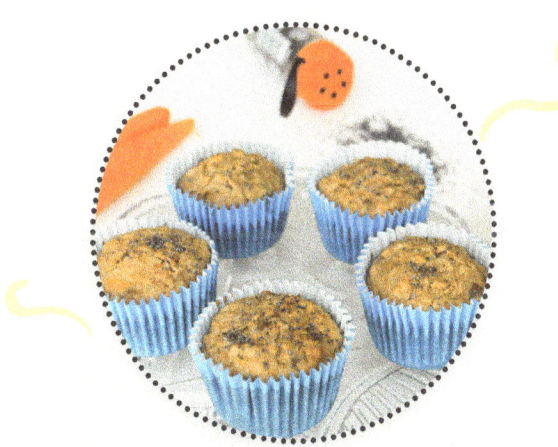

Banana, Honey and Hazelnut Smoothie

PREPARATION 10 MINUTES | SERVES 2

INGREDIENTS:

1 banana, sliced

Soya milk (250ml)

Honey (1 teaspoon)

Ground nutmeg (half a teaspoon)

Hazelnuts (2 teaspoons), chopped and toasted

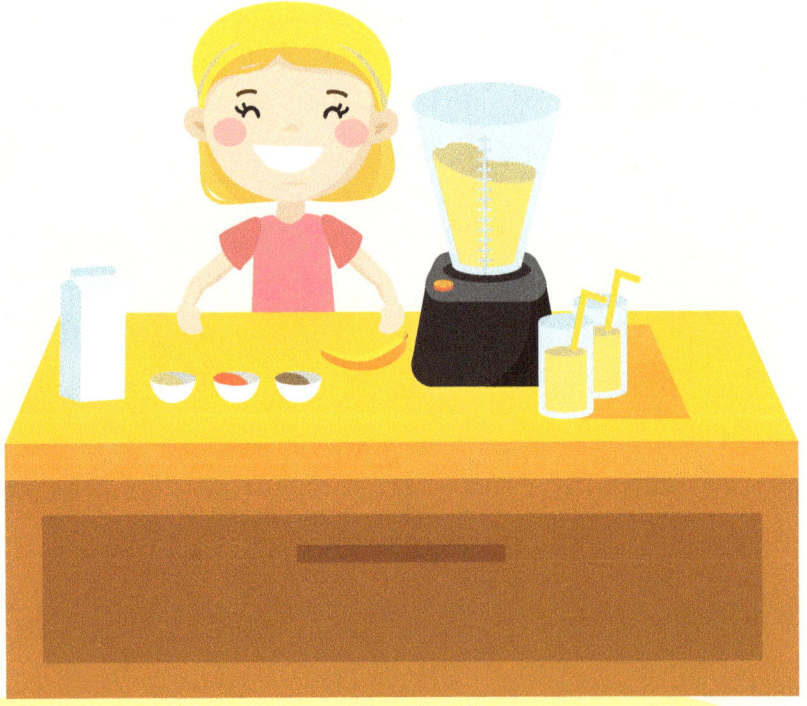

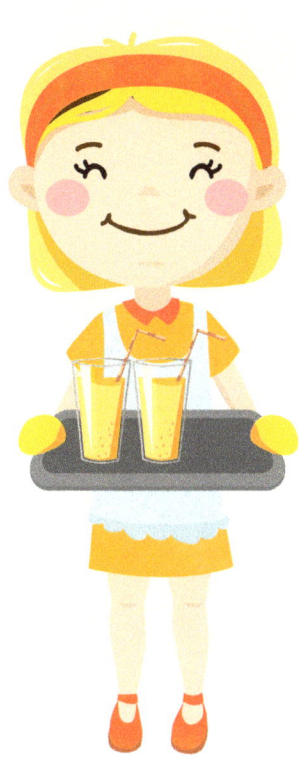

METHOD:

1. Put the banana, soya milk, honey and nutmeg in a smoothie maker or blender. Blend until smooth.
2. Pour into two large glasses and top with the hazelnuts to serve.

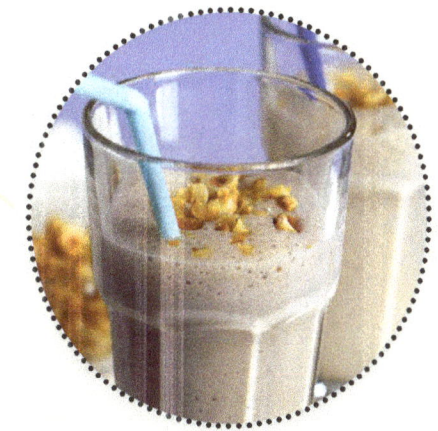

TIPS

If you have a sore mouth or problems chewing, leave out the hazelnuts. Try using finely grated chocolate instead.

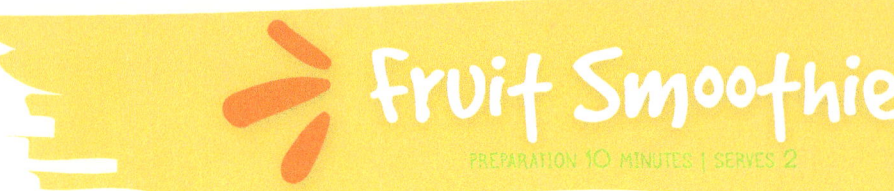

Fruit Smoothie

PREPARATION 10 MINUTES | SERVES 2

Ingredients:

1 tin of peaches or other tinned fruit (400g/14oz), drained

Double cream (150ml/0.25 pint)

Thick and creamy yoghurt (175g/6oz)

Ice-cream (1 scoop)

Apple juice (400ml/0.75 pint)

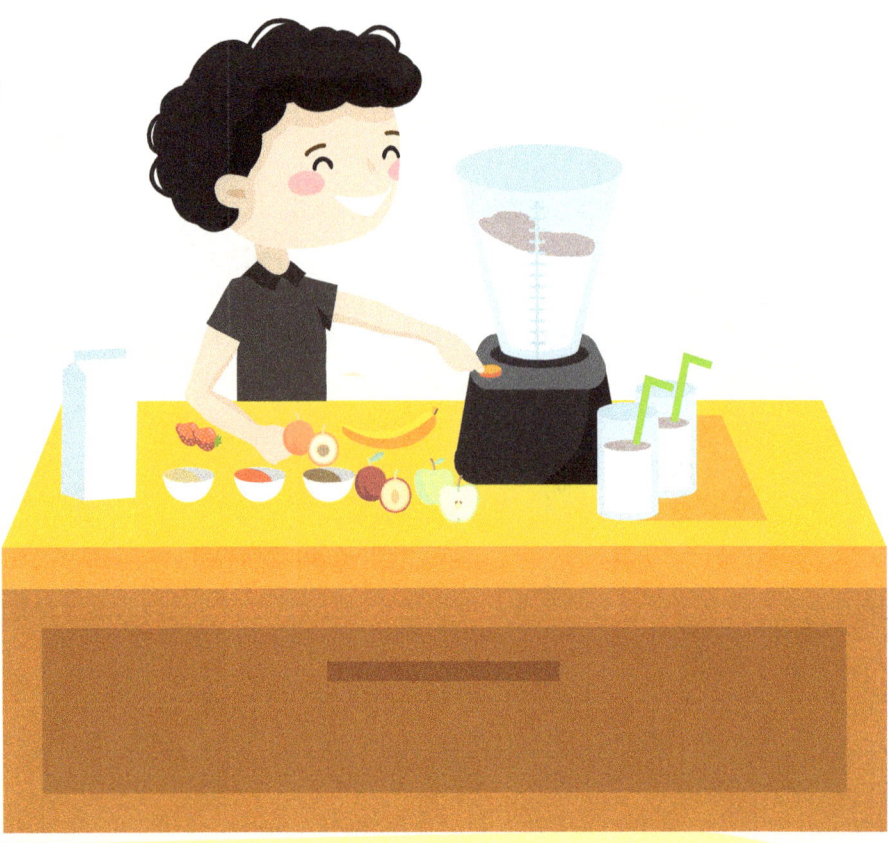

Page 14 MONSTER FIGHTING Recipes

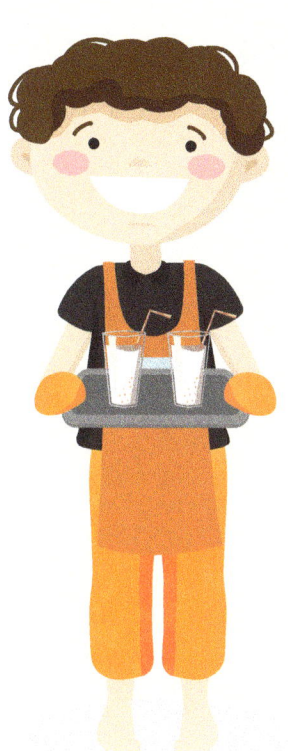

Method:

1. Put all the ingredients in a smoothie maker or blender. Blend until smooth.
2. Serve immediately.

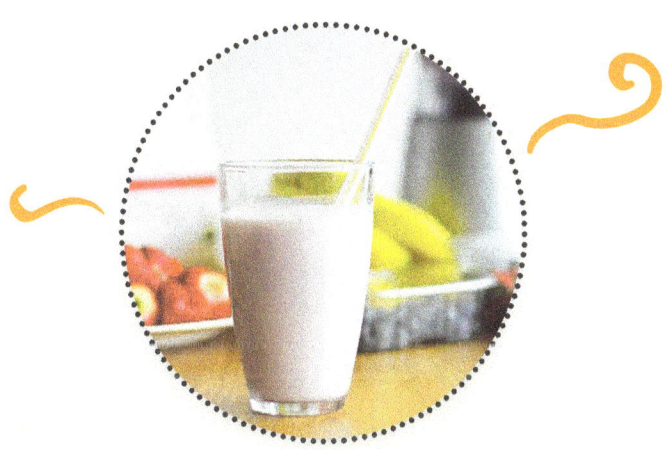

Macmillan Coco Hahona

PREPARATION 5 MINUTES | SERVES 1

Ingredients:

3 chunks of fresh pineapple

1 passion fruit, sliced in half

Passion fruit cordial (3 teaspoons)

Lime juice (4 teaspoons)

Ice, one handful

Coconut water (100ml)

Pineapple leaves, to garnish (optional)

Two round slices of pineapple

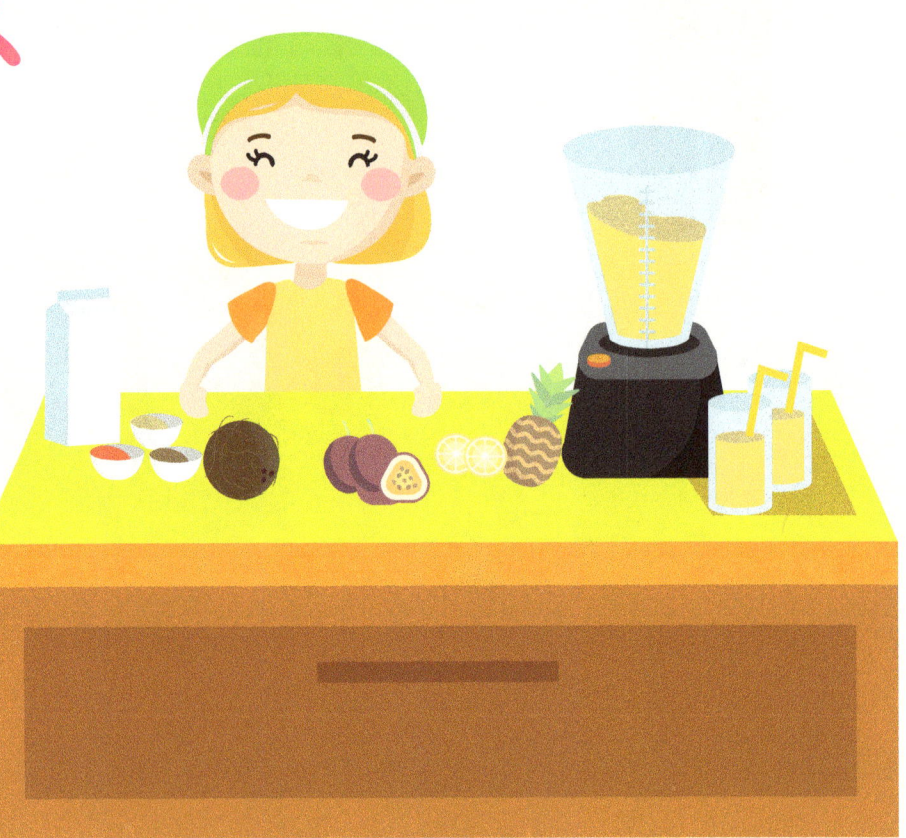

Page 16 MONSTER FIGHTING RECIPES

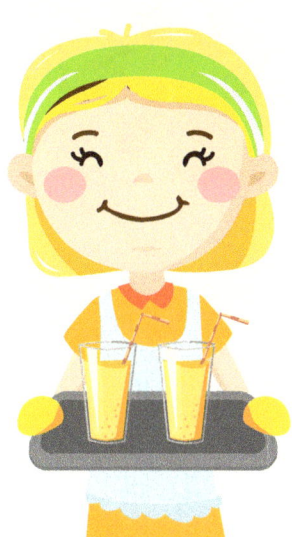

Method:

1. Put the pineapple into a cocktail shaker and scoop in the seeds and flesh from one half of the passion fruit. Crush with a muddler or mix in a blender.
2. 2 Add the passion fruit cordial and lime juice.
3. 3 Add the ice and coconut water, then shake.
4. 4 Pour into a glass and garnish with two round slices of pineapple, the other half of a passion fruit and pineapple leaves.

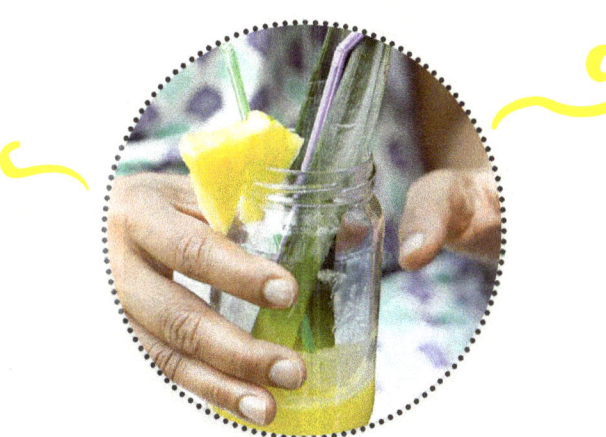

TIPS

You can watch a video of this mocktail being made at gosober.org.uk/blogs/wellbeing/mocktails

Lemon Seeded Muffins

MAKES APPROX 6

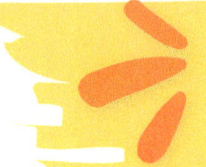

You will need:

6 free range eggs

60ml cup ghee, Coconut Oil or *home-made vegan butter (see recipe in snacks & extras section)

200g coconut flour

120ml cup coconut milk/hemp/almond milk of your choice

60g monkfruit raw extract/sweetener (or stevia)

50ml chamomile or calendula tea steeped overnight

1 tsp vanilla bean seeds

1 tbsp each of lemon juice and lemon zest

1 tbsp each of basil seeds and poppy seeds (soaked overnight in water)

1 tbsp baking powder

1 tsp Ceylon cinnamon

1/2 tsp sea salt

START YOUR DAY WITH THESE SWEET-TASTING, FRESH AND HEALTHY MUFFINS FULL OF GOODNESS.

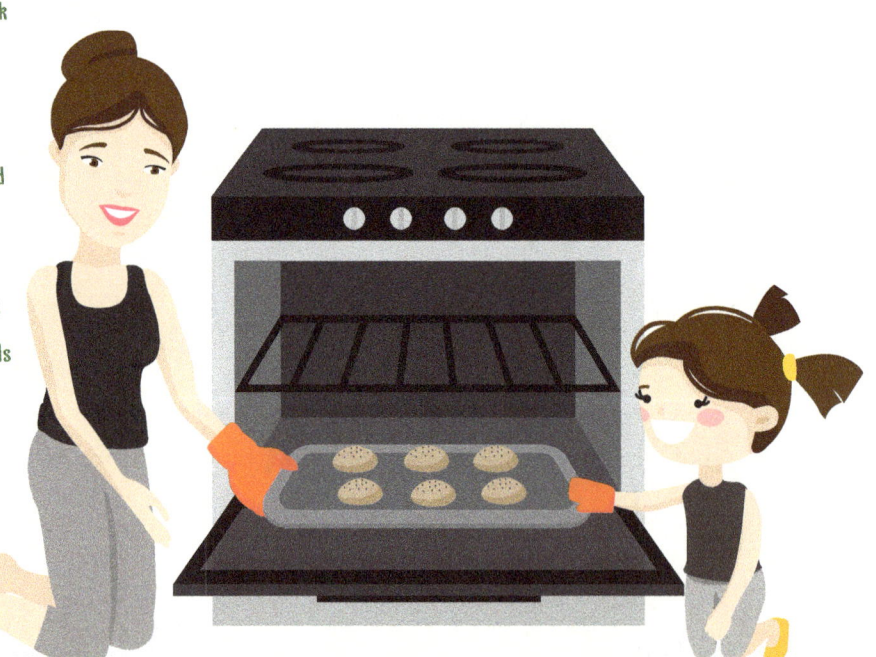

Page 18 MONSTER FIGHTING Recipes

TO MAKE: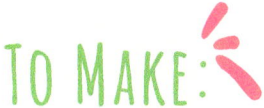

1. Preheat oven to 375F, and line the tin or muffin cases
2. Slice 1/2 a vanilla bean down the centre and scrape out 1 tsp of vanilla seeds
3. Blend the eggs, melted oil/butter, milk, monkfruit, vanilla, basil seeds, poppy seeds, and lemon juice
4. In another bowl blend the dry You will need of coconut flour, cinnamon, salt, baking powder, and lemon zest.
5. Combine You will need together
6. Sit mixture for 5 minutes
7. Transfer mixture to muffin cases
8. Bake for 30 minutes. Cool and store in an air-tight container.

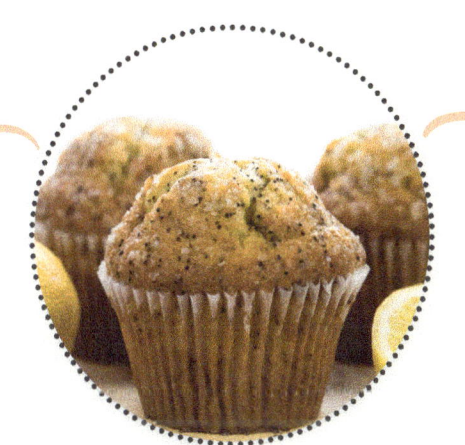

NUTRITIONAL VALUE:

High in fibre, full of protein and healthy fats. Contains selenium, Vitamins A, B1, B2, B6, B9, B12, C, D, Calcium and minerals and trace minerals such as magnesium, potassium, manganese, phosphorus, zinc, iron and copper.

This recipe has anti-bacterial properties, anti-oxidant and anti-inflammatory properties, anti-fungal, anti-diabetic and anti-cancer properties. Helps boost immunity, with calming effects aiding stress reduction and promoting better sleep.

Choc, Vanilla & Cinnamon Smoothie

YOU WILL NEED:

500ml hemp / almond / coconut milk

1 small avocado

1 tsp vanilla pod

1 tsp black seed honey

1 tsp cacao powder / or 100% organic cocoa powder unsweetened

1/2 tsp ceylon cinnamon

1/2 cup crushed ice

A DREAMY MIX OF SIMPLE BUT NOURISHING INGREDIENTS, WITH ITS RICH NUTRITIONAL VALUE. GREAT AT ANY TIME OF THE DAY, AND PERFECT IF YOU NEED SOMETHING LIGHT BUT FILLING.

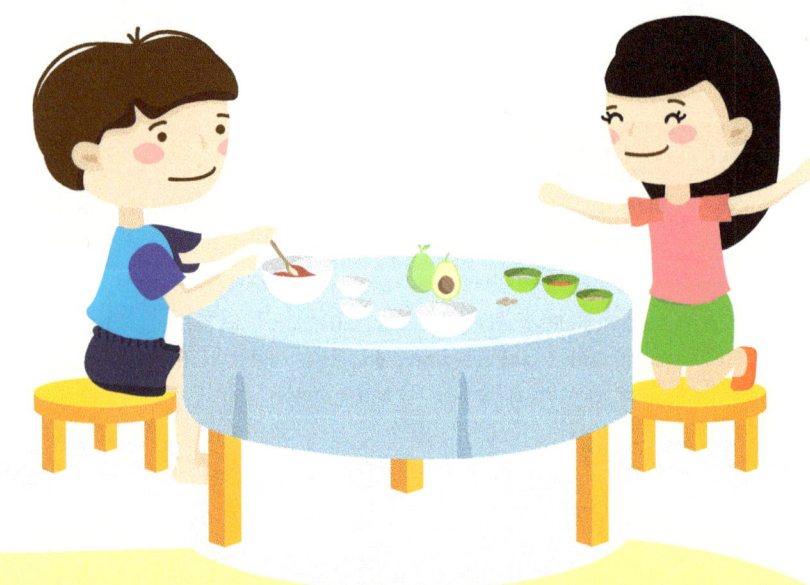

Page 20 MONSTER FIGHTING RECIPES

TO MAKE:

1. Blend avocado, and milk until a velvet smooth paste.
2. Add the vanilla pod seeds by cutting down the middle of the pod and scraping out the seeds, black seed honey, cinnamon and cacao/cocoa powder
3. Finally add the crushed ice and blend just to mix
4. Serve immediately, and top with some almonds if you desire.

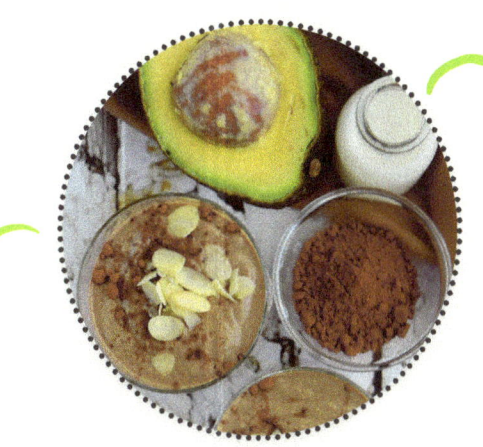

NUTRITIONAL VALUE:

Offering nearly 20 vitamins as well as minerals and trace minerals such as, potassium, magnesium, Zinc, Iron, Phosphorus, Calcium, Copper and Manganese. High in Protein, Fibre and antioxidants. An Energy and immune boosting recipe, with ingredients that help to support the respiratory, and digestive system. Supporting symptoms such as stomach ulcers, liver ailments, diseases due to malnutrition, eye diseases, surgical wounds and a host of other issues. We have included ingredients that offer natural antibacterial and antibiotic properties, calm the body's nervous system, anti-inflammatory, anti-fungal, and anti-diabetic properties.

Celery Juice

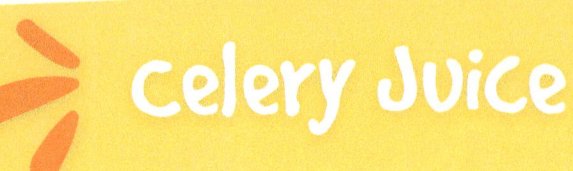

You will need:

1 packet of organic celery

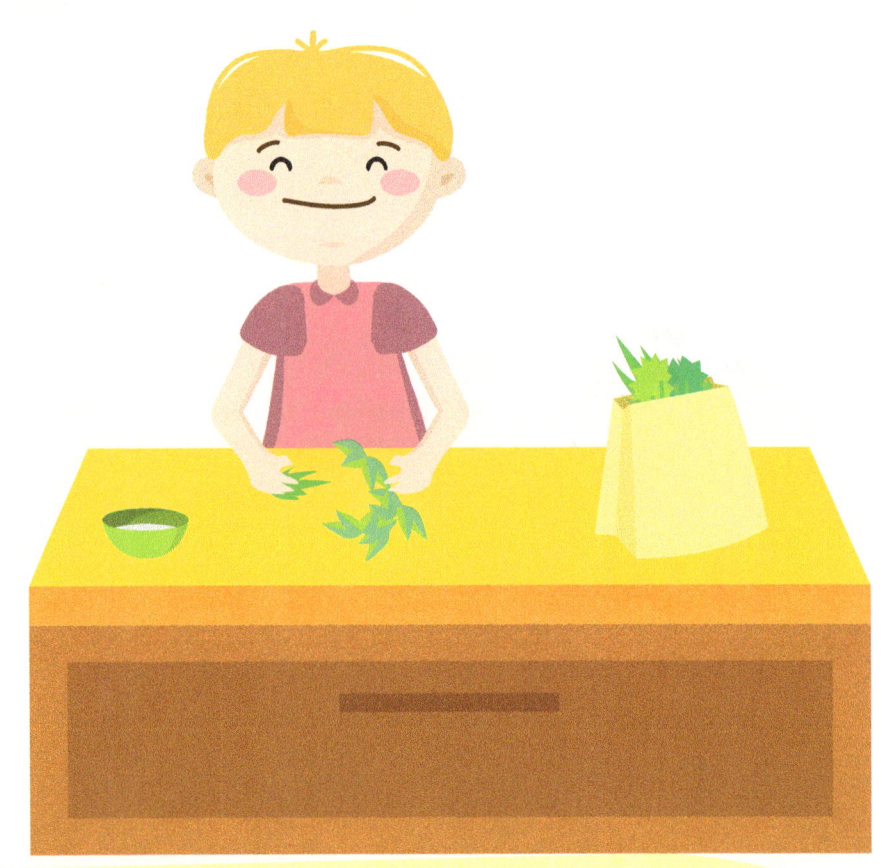

Page 22 MONSTER FIGHTING Recipes

How to Make:

1. Scrub the celery well
2. Add the celery into a bowl of filtered water with 1 tsp bicarbonate of soda, soak for 12 minutes
3. Replace with clean filtered water and soak for 2 minutes
4. Now the stalks are clean and ready to use
5. Add into the juicer
6. Serve

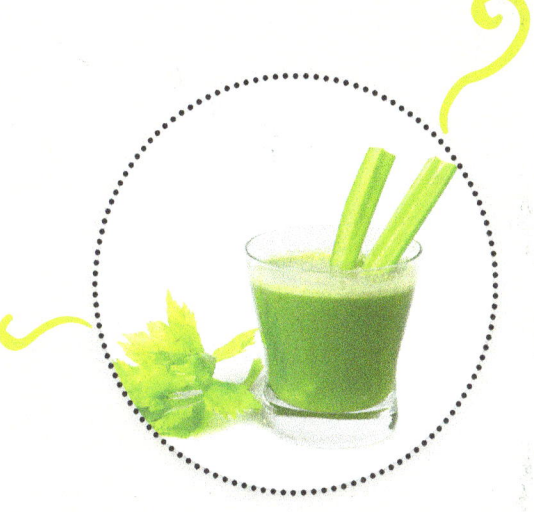

Nutritional Value:

Celery is rich in vitamin K, and it also contains Vitamin A and B9, C, potassium. Celery is mainly water, but it is also a good source of dietary fibre. Celery acts as a natural anti-inflammatory due to its flavonoids, and antioxidant properties. It has numerous amazing benefits for skin, liver, eye and cognitive health, and drinking celery juice each morning on an empty stomach can help kill off unwanted visitors.

Toasted Cinnamon and Vanilla Nuts

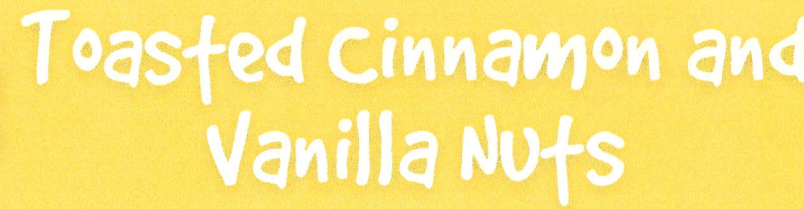

You will need:

250g mixture of selected nuts – almonds / cashews / pecans / hickory etc

1-2 tsp ceylon cinnamon

1-2 tsp vanilla pod or raw black seed honey

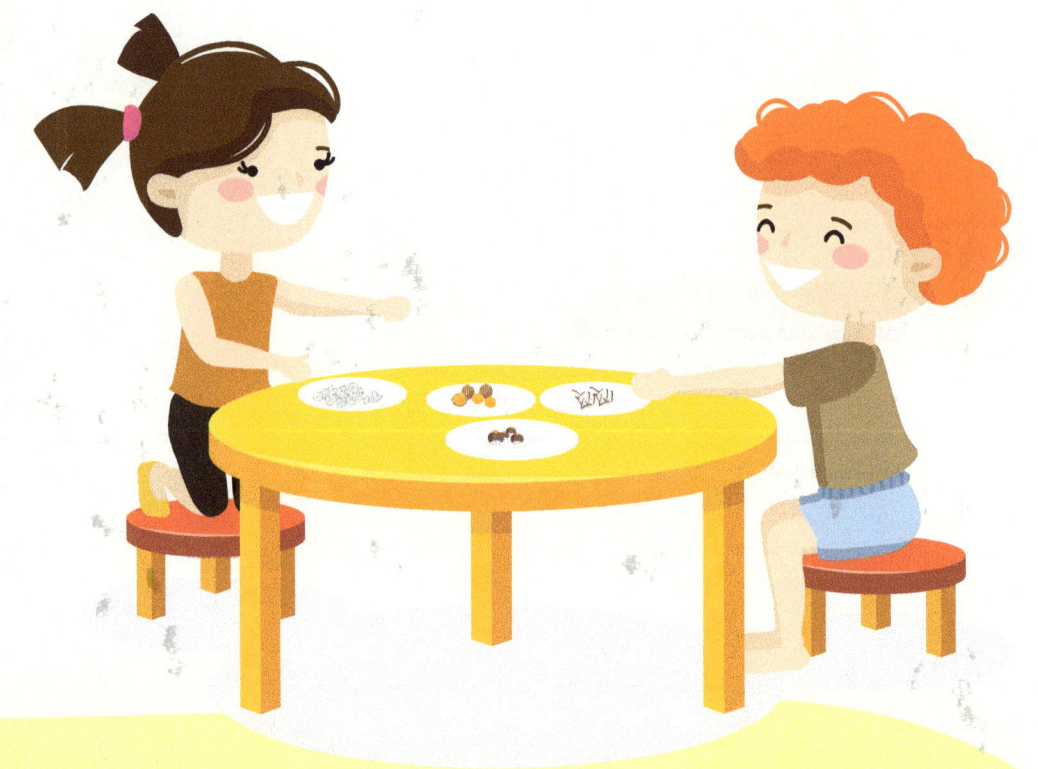

How To Make:

1. Place nuts into a bowl and add 2 tsp cinnamon and 1 tsp vanilla pod
2. Distribute the seasoning to the nuts
3. Add onto a tray on baking paper
4. Place in preheated oven 180°C for 15 minutes

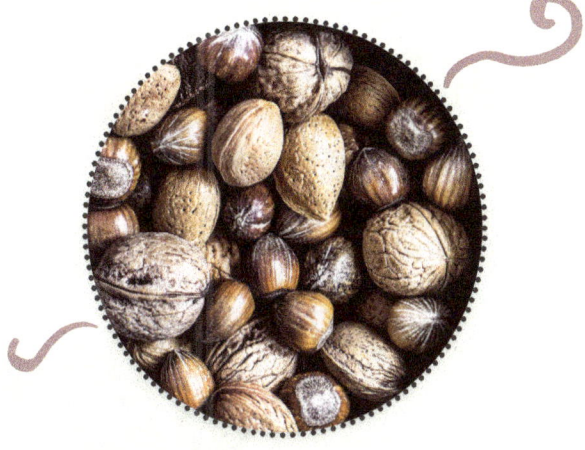

NUTRITIONAL VALUE:

Rich in vitamin E, calcium, magnesium, zinc, copper, potassium, and manganese - which helps protect cells from oxidative stress, help maintain strong bones, build connective tissue, and contribute to normal energy-yielding metabolism. This recipe is a significant source of protein and fibre. A metabolic health boost, with good fats and may contain anti-inflammatory properties.

Full of anti-oxidants, anti-fungal, anti-diabetic and immune boosting properties.

Pecan and Hazelnut Bread

A NOURISHING, NUTRITIOUS AND TASTY GRAIN FREE BREAD WITH A SOFT TEXTURE AND EASY TO MAKE

You will need:

- 4 eggs
- 200g high quality blanched (skins removed) almond flour
- 100g of ground pecans and hazelnuts
- 2 tbsp soaked pumpkin seeds
- 4 tbsp flaxseed meal
- 6 tbsp arrowroot powder
- 2 tsp coconut flour
- 2 tbsp tapioca starch
- 100ml unsweetened hemp, coconut or almond milk (add more if needed)
- 1 tsp bicarbonate soda
- 1 tbsp olive oil
- 1 tbsp apple cider vinegar
- 1/2 tsp sea salt

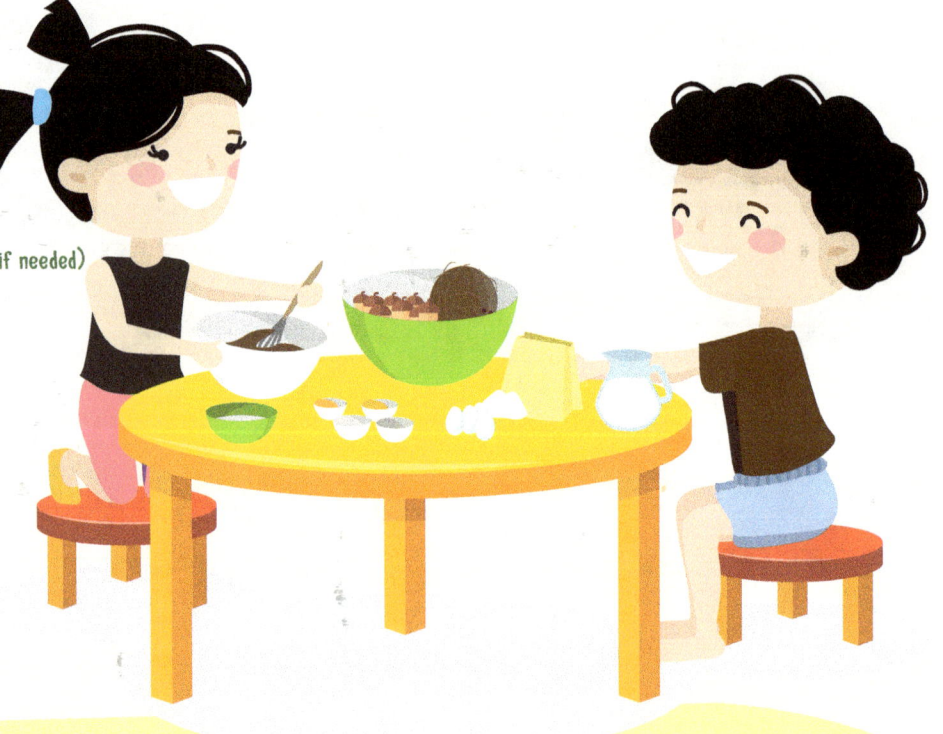

How to Make:

1. Mix all of the dry ingredients together, then add the eggs, olive oil, water and apple cider vinegar. Blend until smooth then add to a lined tin
2. Place in the oven on 200C for 30-40 minutes or until golden and centre knife/cocktail stick test comes out clean
3. Remove from oven and dish to cool.

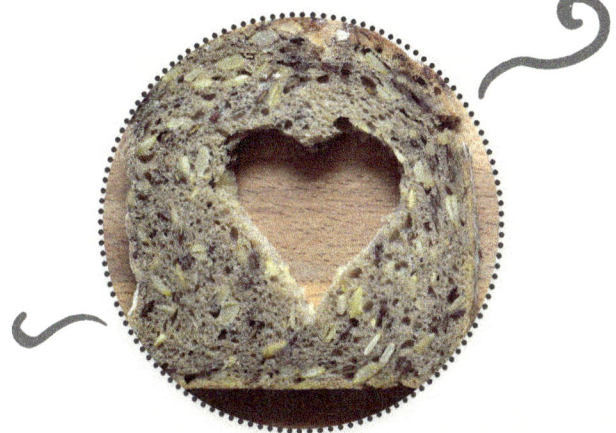

NUTRITIONAL VALUE:

Full of protein and fibre, Vitamins B2, B6, B12, D, E, K, minerals and trace minerals such as iron, calcium, magnesium, selenium, potassium and zinc, copper and manganese – these last two minerals that help to boost overall metabolic health, and may contain anti-inflammatory and anti-bacterial properties. Rich in unsaturated fats (mostly oleic acid), omega-3's, and omega-6's, the nuts and seeds are good for your heart, can help reduce the risk of cancer, and aid in muscle, skin, bone, joint and digestive health and diabetes. Studies have even shown that arrowroot can stimulate immune cells and boost the immune system.

Beginner's Luck

DESCRIPTION:

The Beginner's Luck Green Smoothie is a great beginner friendly green smoothie recipe. It's full of iron, potassium and vitamins galore— AND tastes like a tropical treat from all the island fruit.

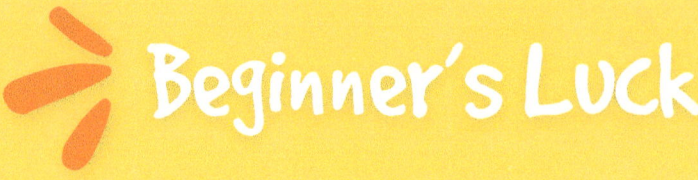

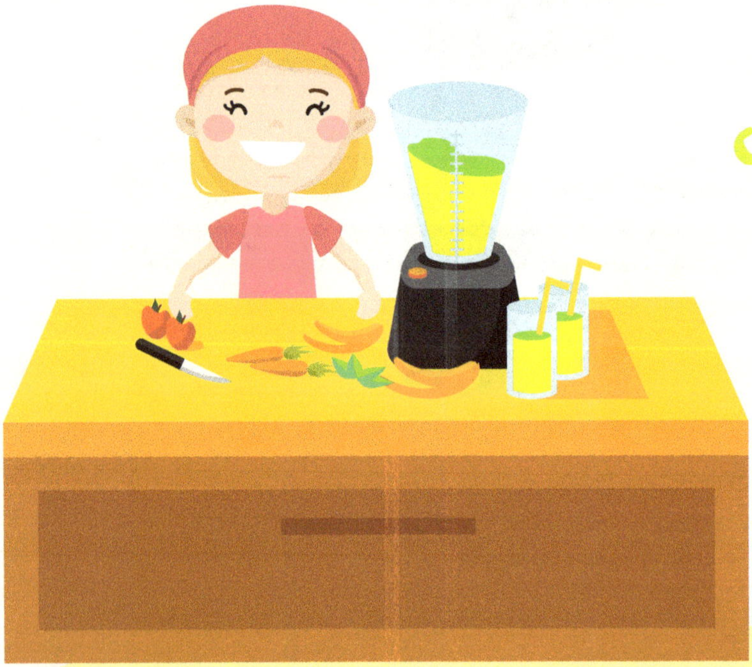

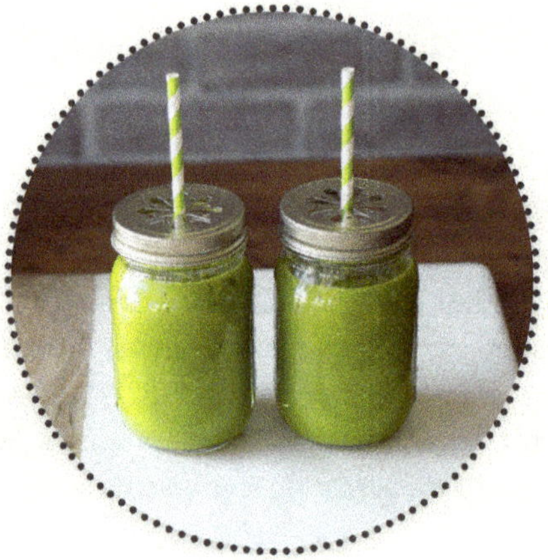

Page 28 Monster Fighting Recipes

INGREDIENTS:

1 cup spinach (fresh)
1 cup water
1/2 cup pineapple
1/2 cup mango
1 banana (peeled)*

*Not a fan of bananas? Swap it for 1/4 avocado or add another 1/2 cup mango to the recipe.

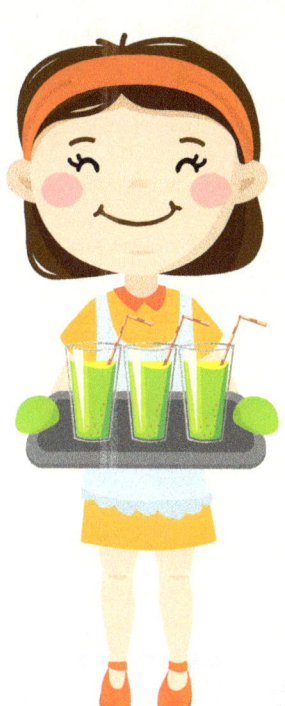

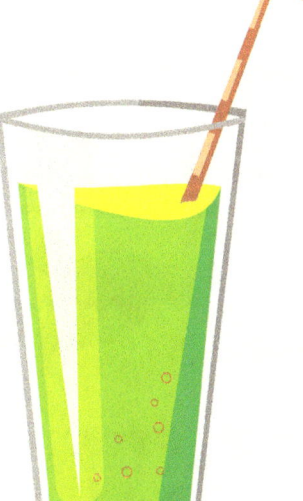

INSTRUCTIONS:

1. Tightly pack spinach in a measuring cup.
2. Add spinach to blender with water. Blend together until all chunks are gone. (Should resemble green water when blended well).
3. Add pineapple, mango and banana to blender. I like to use frozen pineapple and mangos to chill the smoothie down and save time cutting and prepping. It's a win-win!
4. Blend all together until smooth and creamy. Depending on your blender, this could take as little as 30 seconds or as long as 2 minutes.
5. Pour into a glass and serve immediately.
6. You can also store the smoothie in the fridge with a lid until ready to drink.

Carrot, Apple and Sultana Muffins

MAKES 12 MUFFINS

Ingredients:

175g (6 oz) self-raising flour

1 tsp ground ginger

1 tsp ground cinnamon

1 tsp bicarbonate of soda

100g (3 1/2 oz) light brown sugar

2 eggs

3 tbsp golden syrup

150 ml (1/4 pint) sunflower oil

150g (5 oz) carrots, peeled and grated

50g (2 oz) apple, peeled, cored and grated

75g (3 oz) sultanas

One of my favourite muffins and they are quick and easy to prepare. You could make 24 mini muffins instead. Simply chop the sultanas in half before mixing and bake for about 12 minutes.

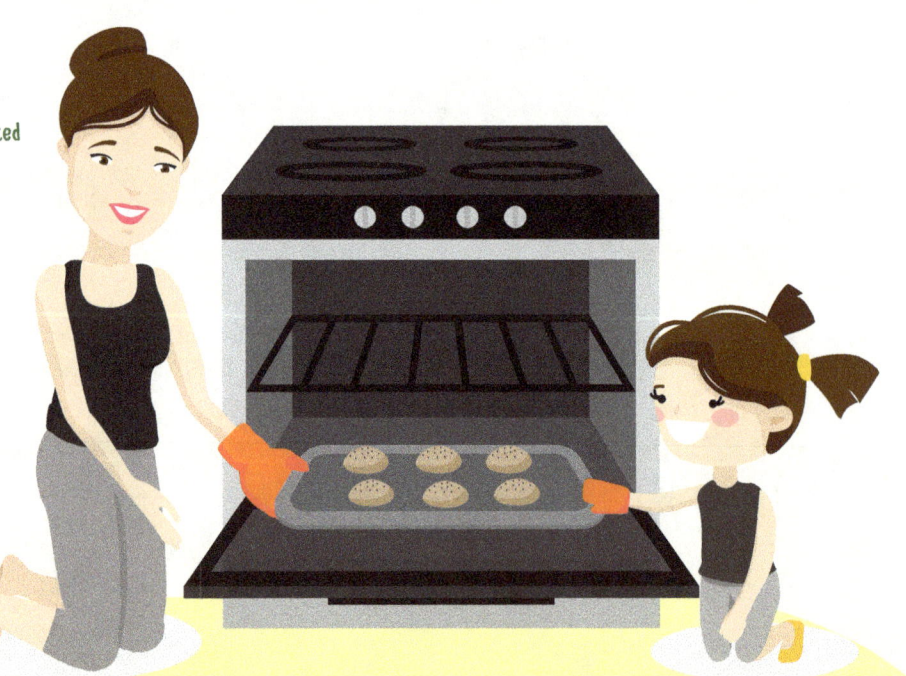

Page 30 Monster Fighting Recipes

Method: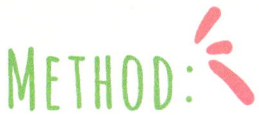

1. Preheat the oven to 200 C / 400 F Gas 6. Line a muffin tin with paper cases.
2. Sift the flour, spices and bicarbonate of soda into a bowl, then add the sugar. In a separate bowl, combine the eggs, golden syrup and oil, then pour them into the bowl with the dry ingredients. Whisk until smooth. Stir in the carrot, apple and sultanas.
3. Spoon the mixture into the muffin cases. Bake for about 20 to 22 minutes, until the muffins are well risen and golden brown.
4. Allow the muffins to cool in the tin for about ~10 minutes, then transfer to a wire rack to cool completely. Store in an airtight container

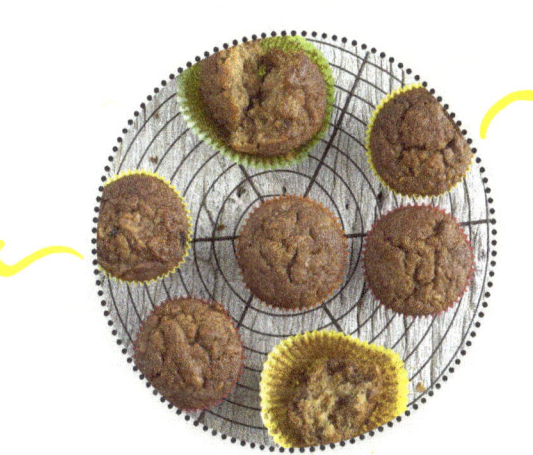

Butternut Squash, Leek and Parmesan Risotto

PREPARATION 15 MINUTES | COOKING 35 MINUTES | SERVES 3

Ingredients:

Olive oil (2 tablespoons)

Butternut squash (400g), cut into small chunks

Arborio rice (300g)

1 leek, thinly sliced

Vegetable stock (1.2 litres/2 pints)

Fresh thyme (1 tablespoon), chopped

Lemon zest (1 teaspoon), finely grated

Frozen peas (80g)

Parmesan cheese (4 tablespoons), finely grated

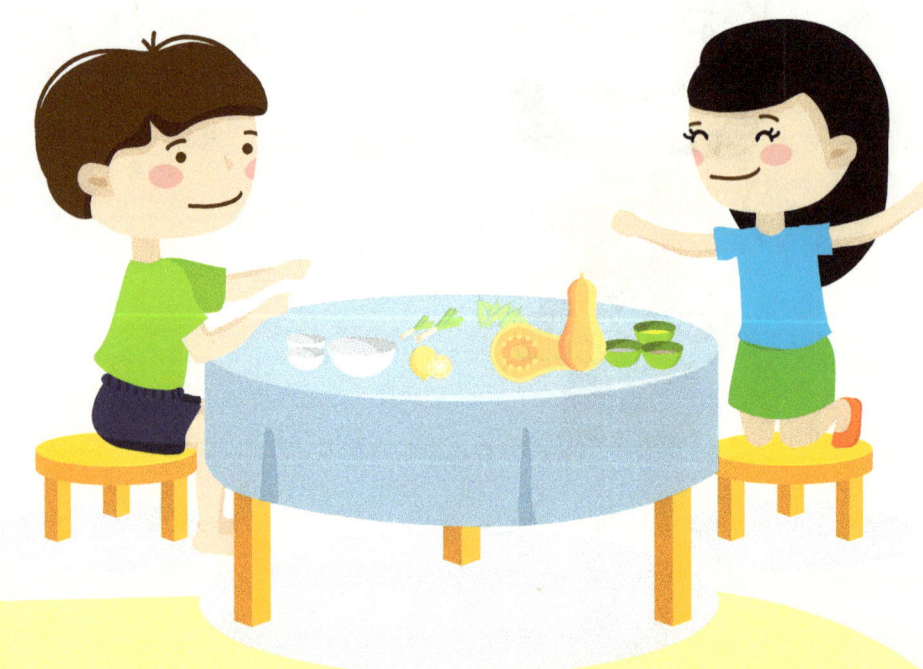

Method: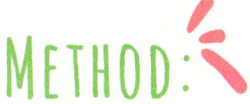

1. Heat the oil in a large pan. Add the butternut squash and rice. Gently fry for 1 to 2 minutes. Stir in the leek.
2. Add about a third of the stock. Cook over a low heat, stirring often, until the liquid has almost been absorbed.
3. Gradually add the remaining stock, cooking gently for 25 to 30 minutes until the liquid has been absorbed and the rice is tender.
4. Add the thyme, lemon zest and peas. Cook for 2 to 3 minutes, then stir in half the parmesan.
5. Sprinkle with the rest of the parmesan, then serve.

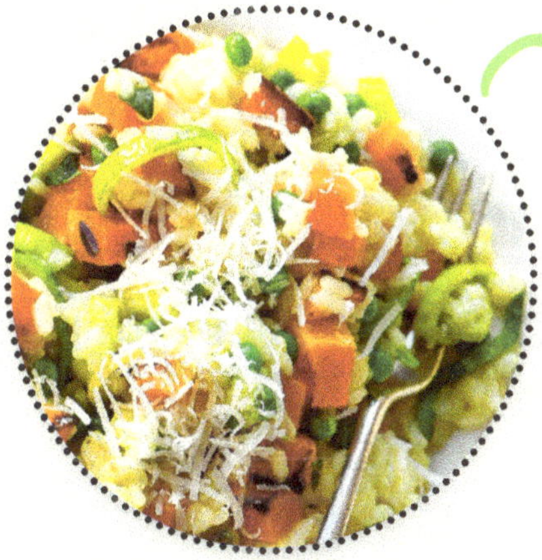

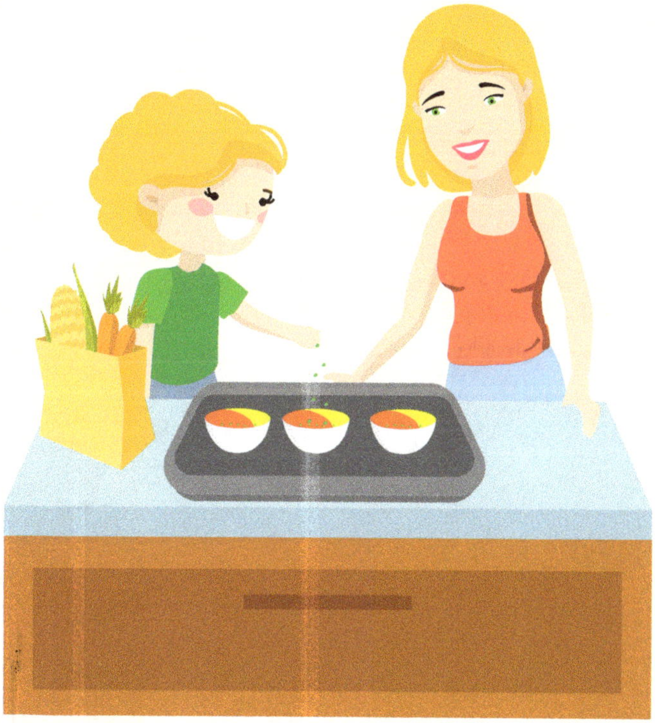

TIPS

Use a spray oil in a non-stick pan to reduce the fat content.

Vegetable Leather

You will need:

2 cups fresh pumpkin, cooked and puréed with a little lemon juice

4 tbsp black seed raw honey

1/4 tsp Ceylon cinnamon

1/8 tsp all-spice

1/8 teaspoon nutmeg

1/8 teaspoon powdered cloves

(for a slightly more firmer texture you could add 1/8 teaspoon of agar agar – vegetable glycerine). Agar agar is made from seaweed.

A SWEET TREAT WITH NO ARTIFICIAL SUGAR

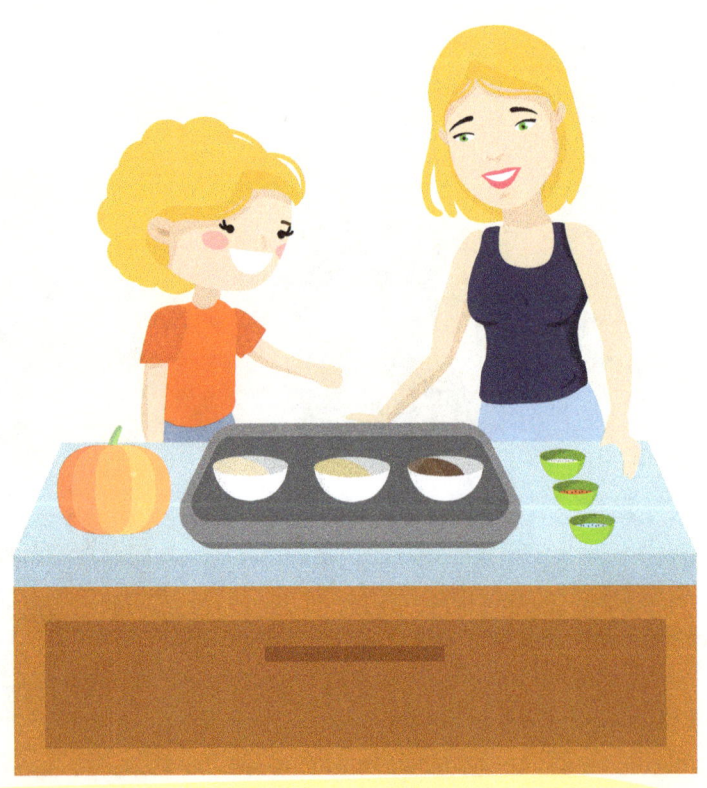

How To Make:

1. Blend ingredients well. Spread on a tray lined with parchment paper 1/4 inch thick. Dry at 120-140°C for 6-8 hours, or until the leather is not sticky and can be rolled. Remove from oven. Cool and roll up between parchment paper to store.

2. Will store for 1 month in a container or freeze to store for up to 1 year.

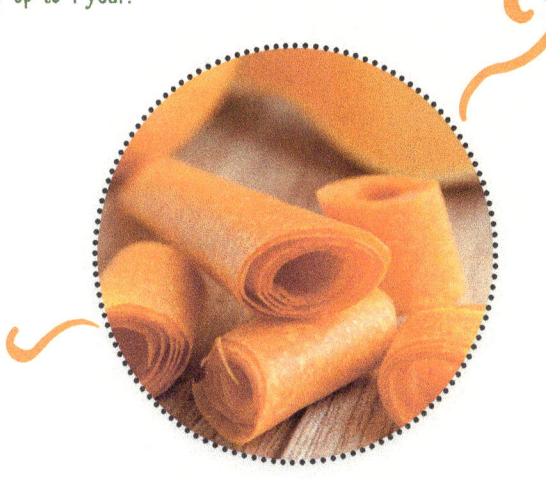

NUTRITIONAL VALUE:

Great source of Vitamins A, C, B1, B6, B9, B12, E, Iron, Magnesium, Calcium and Phosphorus, and a very good source of Fibre, Potassium, Copper and Manganese. Its nutrients and antioxidants may help to boost your immune system, protect your eyesight, lower your risk of certain cancers and promote heart and skin health. With ingredients that act as a natural antibacterial, antiseptic and antibiotic agent, full of anti-oxidants, anti-inflammatory and pain relieving properties, anti-fungal, anti-diabetic, analgesic, antipyretic, anticancer, and anti-tumorigenic properties, this recipe is powerful and healing.

Page 36 Monster Fighting Recipes

LIGHT LUNCH

Lil' Adventurer Cauliflower Smoothie Bowl

DESCRIPTION:

Yep! We've blended cauliflower with some of our favorite fruits to create a tasty + nutrient-packed smoothie bowl to fuel you for you adventures ahead. I made this recipe for the lil' adventurers out there like my son Jackson... and those of us that have grown up and are still adventurers at heart.

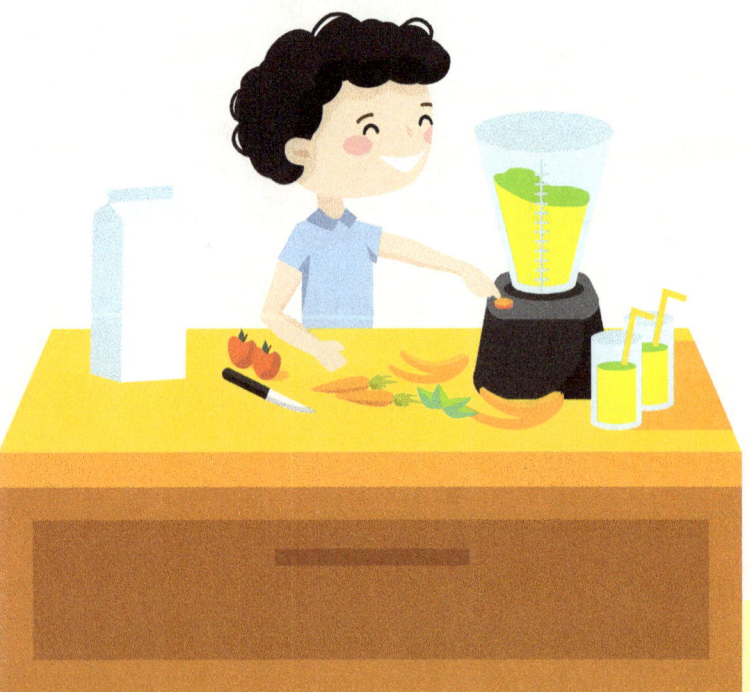

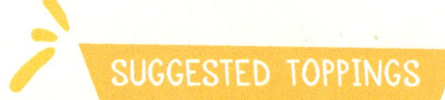

SUGGESTED TOPPINGS

Strawberries

Blueberries

Kiwi

INGREDIENTS:

1/4 cup carrots (raw)
1/4 cup cauliflower florets (frozen)
1 large orange (peeled)
1 large banana (frozen)
1/2 cup pineapple (frozen)

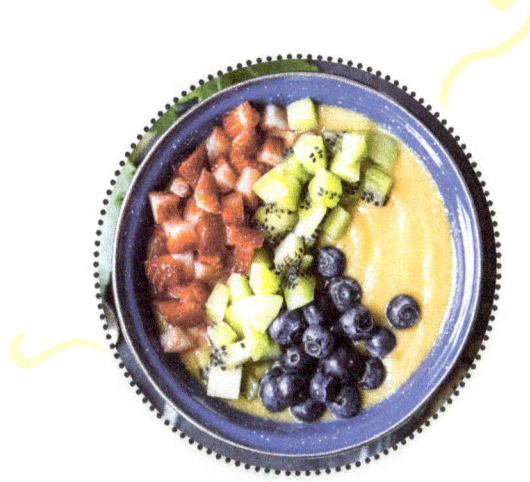

INSTRUCTIONS:

1. Blend carrots, cauliflower, orange, banana and pineapple all ingredients together. You may need to use a tamper, if it's hard to blend on it's own. (You do want this to be thicker than a smoothie, since it's a smoothie bowl.)
2. Pour blended ingredients into a bowl and top with your fav fresh fruits. We used blueberries, strawberries and kiwi for this one today.

Caribbean-Style Tuna Spread

PREPARATION 15 MINUTES | SERVES 2

Ingredients:

2 tins of tuna (200g each), drained

1 small red onion, finely diced

1 spring onion, chopped

1 small stalk of celery, finely diced

Cucumber (4 tablespoons), finely diced

1 red or yellow pepper, finely diced (optional)

Black pepper

Caribbean hot pepper sauce (half a teaspoon) (optional)

Mayonnaise (1 tablespoon)

Half an avocado, diced

Lemon juice (1 and a half teaspoons)

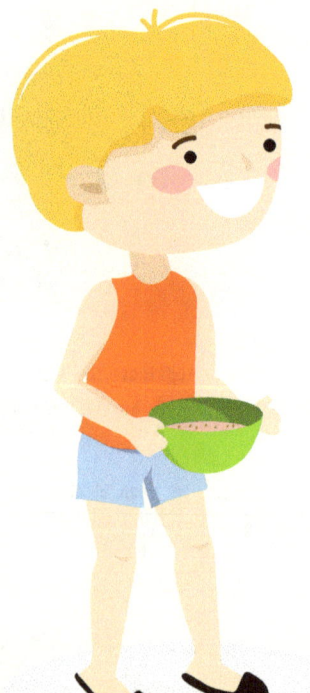
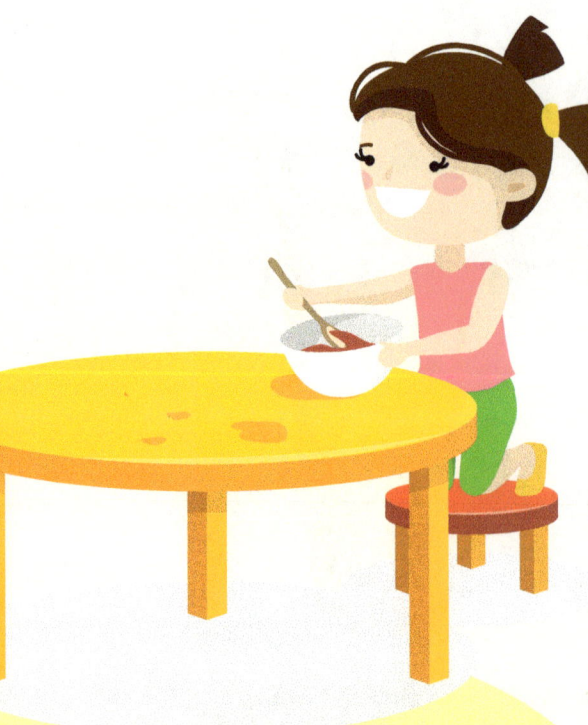

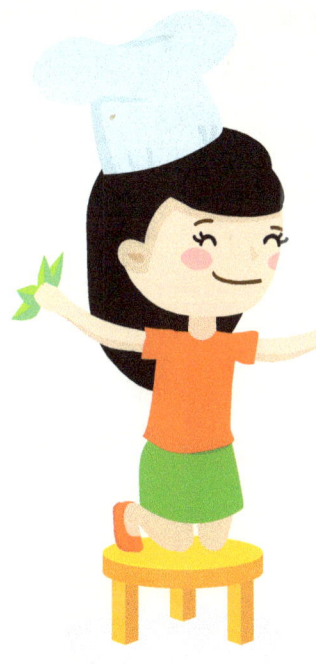

Method:

1. Open the tins of tuna and squeeze the liquid out.
2. Flake the tuna into small pieces in a large bowl. Don't overwork it or it will become mushy.
3. Add all the ingredients, except the avocado and lemon juice. Mix well.
4. Add in the avocado and lemon juice. Gently fold in the avocado, taking care not to crush it.
5. Adjust the seasoning or add more lemon juice to taste.
6. Serve the mixture in a sandwich, on crackers or on a baked potato.

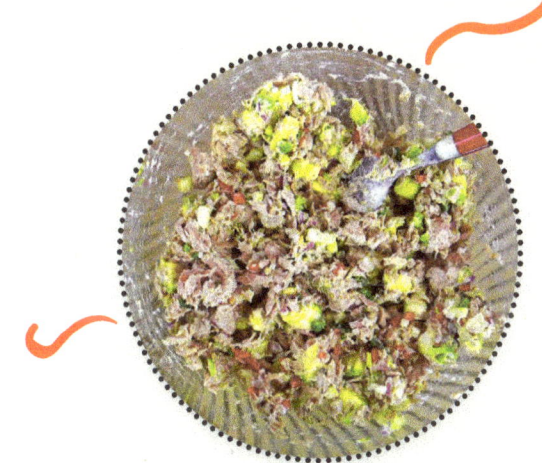

NUTRITIONAL INFORMATION PER PORTION (without bread, crackers or baked potato)

Energy 270kcal, Protein 31.9g, Total fat 14g (of which saturates 2.2g).

Carbohydrate 4.2g, Fibre 2.2g

Sardine bruschetta

PREPARATION 10 MINUTES | COOKING 6 MINUTES | SERVES 4

Ingredients:

1 tin of peeled plum tomatoes (400g), drained and roughly chopped

1 red onion, finely chopped

2 garlic cloves, crushed

Large handful of fresh basil, finely chopped

Olive oil (1 tablespoon)

Salt and black pepper

2 bread rolls

2 tins of sardines in tomato sauce (240g)

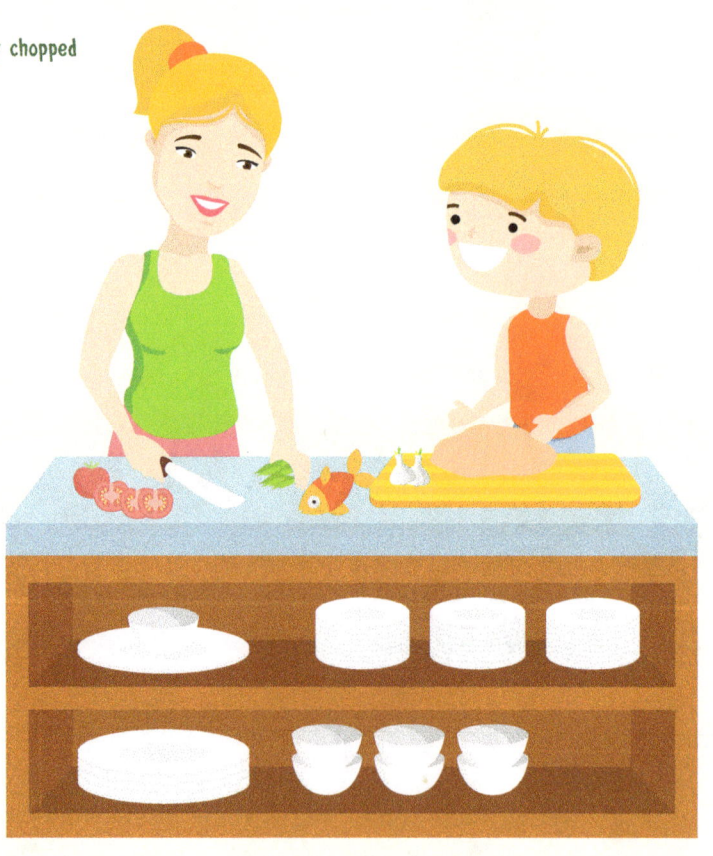

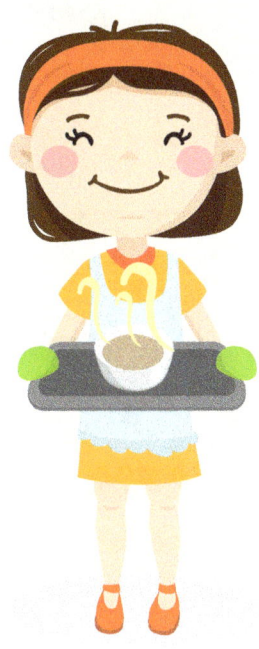

Method:

1. Preheat the oven to 220°C/200°C fan/gas mark 7.
2. Put all the ingredients, except the bread rolls and sardines, in a large bowl. Mix thoroughly.
3. Cut the rolls in half and place in the oven for 2 minutes.
4. Remove the rolls from the oven and spoon the mixture over the top of each roll.
5. Put the sardine fillets on to each roll and place back in the oven for 4 minutes. Serve warm.

TIPS

If you have a dry or sore mouth, try serving the mixture with pasta or on a baked potato instead.

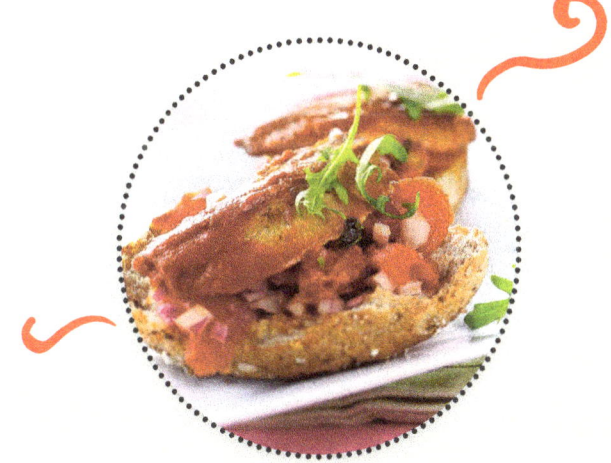

Minty Summer Rice Salad

PREPARATION 5 MINUTES | COOKING 20 MINUTES | SERVES 4

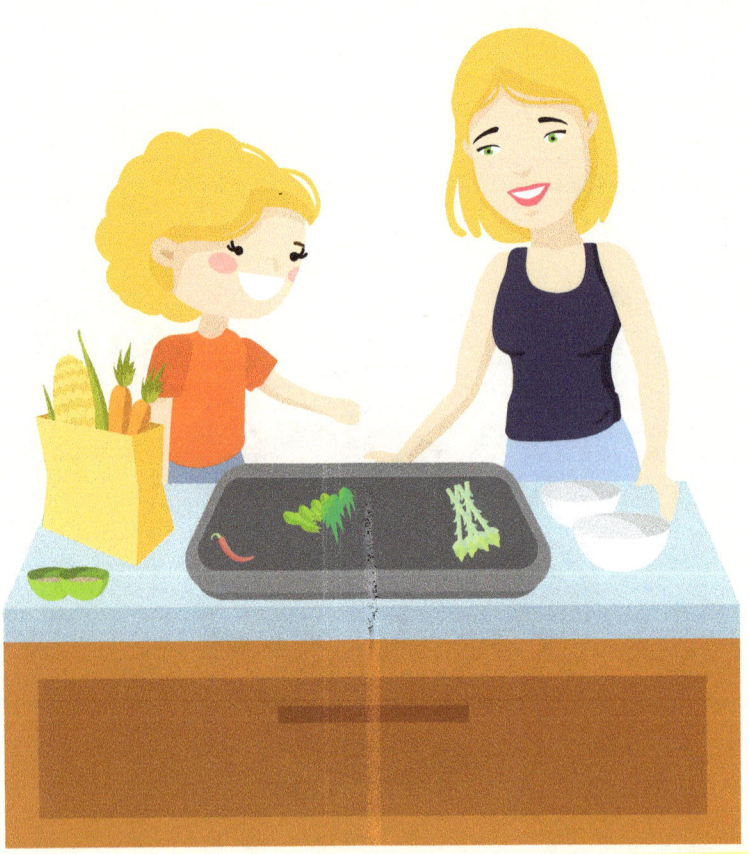

Ingredients:

Long-grain rice (250g)

Asparagus (250g), chopped into bite-sized pieces

1 red pepper, deseeded and chopped

Olive oil (3 tablespoons)

Grated zest and juice of 1 lemon

Mozzarella (250g), cut into small pieces

Large bunch of mint, chopped

Salt and black pepper

Page 46 Monster Fighting Recipes

Method:

1. Add the rice to a pan of boiling, salted water and cook for 10 minutes.
2. 2 Add the asparagus and cook for 3 to 4 minutes until the rice is completely cooked and the asparagus is slightly crunchy.
3. 3 Drain into a sieve and hold under cold, running water until cool.
4. 4 When the rice is cold, stir in the rest of the ingredients.
5. 5 Finish with a pinch of salt and black pepper, then serve.

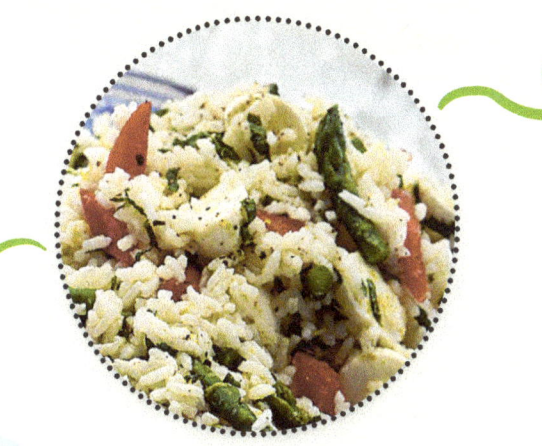

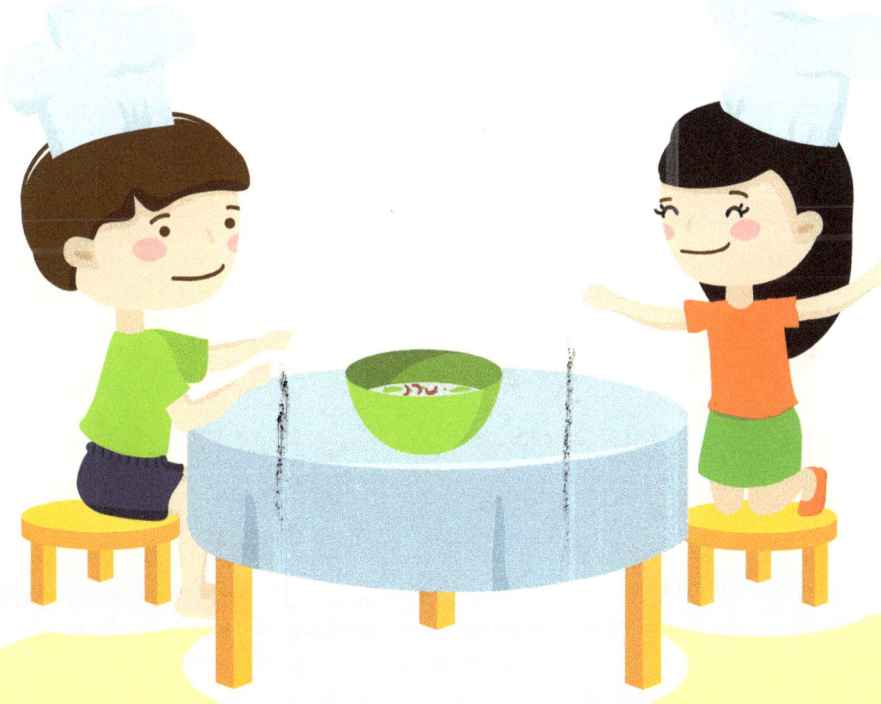

Parsnip and coconut soup

PREPARATION 15 MINUTES | COOKING 45 MINUTES | SERVES 4 TO 6

Ingredients:

Olive oil (2 tablespoons)

1 large onion, chopped

1 garlic clove, finely chopped

Fresh ginger (25mm/1 inch), peeled and chopped

Garam masala (1 tablespoon)

6 parsnips (about 600g), roughly chopped

Full-fat coconut milk (500ml/1 pint)

Vegetable stock (1 litre/2 pints)

Salt and black pepper

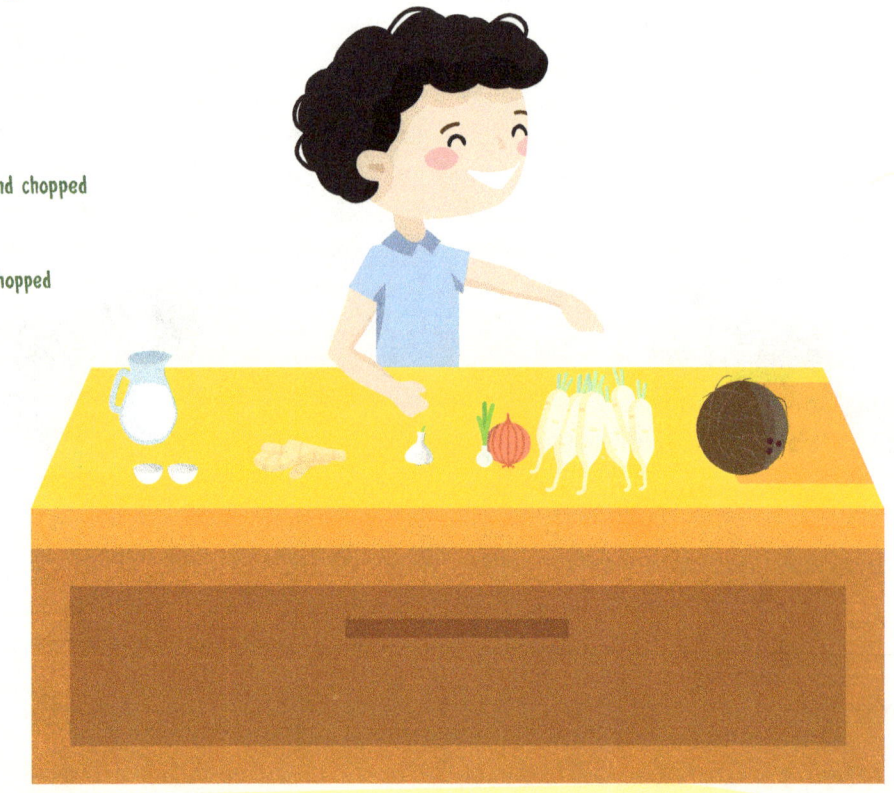

Page 48 MONSTER FIGHTING Recipes

Method: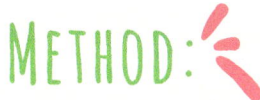

1. Heat the olive oil in a large pan. Add the onion, garlic, ginger and garam masala. Gently fry the mixture for 3 to 5 minutes, until the onions begin to soften but not brown.
2. Add the parsnips and mix well with the other ingredients to bring out all the flavours.
3. Pour the coconut milk and stock into the pan. Season with salt and pepper and bring the soup to the boil. Stir well.
4. Reduce the heat to a gentle simmer and cook with the lid on for 30 minutes.
5. Check the parsnips are soft by piercing through to the centre with a sharp knife. Remove the soup from the heat and blend to a smooth puree with a blender or food processor.
6. Finish with a pinch of salt and black pepper, then serve.

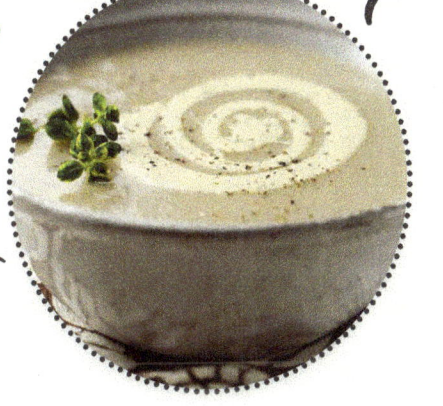

TIPS

To lower the fat content, use low-fat coconut milk.

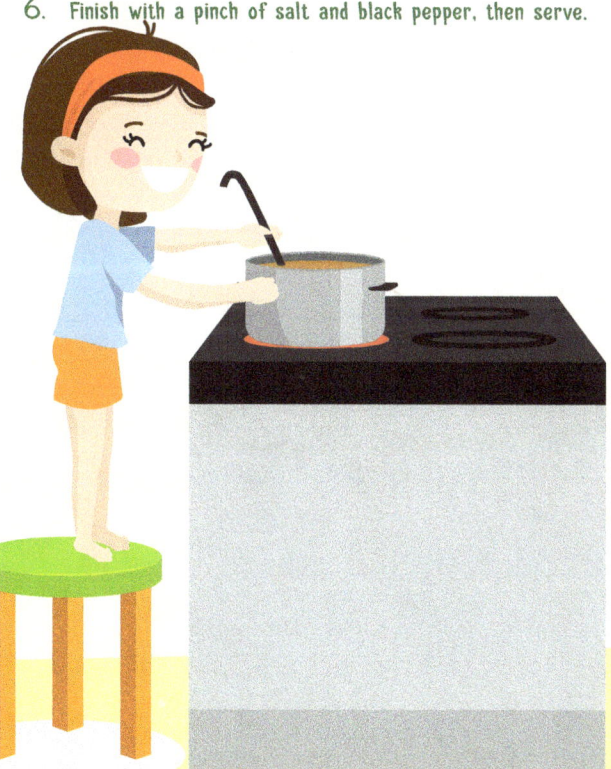

Rainbow oven omelette
MAKES APPROX 4

You will need:

6 x eggs
50ml Dairy free milk
3-4 tablespoon olive oil
1 x shallot
1/2 red pepper, chopped
1/2 yellow pepper, chopped
1/2 cup of petit pois
Small handful of organic spinach
1 inch zucchini, grated
5 shiitake mushrooms, chopped
2 tsp mixed seaweed flakes
Small handful of parsley and coriander, chopped
Small handful thai holy basil
1 tsp celery seeds
1 inch fresh ginger, grated
1 inch turmeric, grated
1 garlic clove, crushed
Pasture Fed Cooked Bacon, chopped small (*optional)

ENJOY THE COLOURFUL VARIETY OF NUTRIENTS THAT THIS DISH BRINGS, AND THE DIFFERENT TASTES TO CREATE A DELICIOUS NUTRITIOUS LUNCH OPTION.

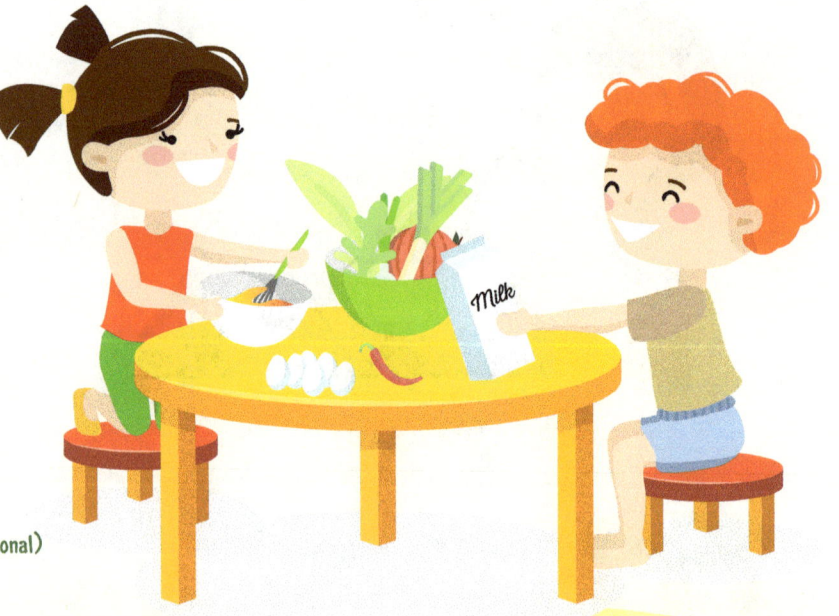

To Make:

1. Preheat the oven to 200°C
2. Mix the eggs, milk and olive oil together in a bowl, until blended
3. Stir in the rest of the ingredients, adding the herbs in last
4. Pour mix into a square baking dish and pop into the oven on 180-200 for 30 minutes or until eggs are cooked and omelette is set

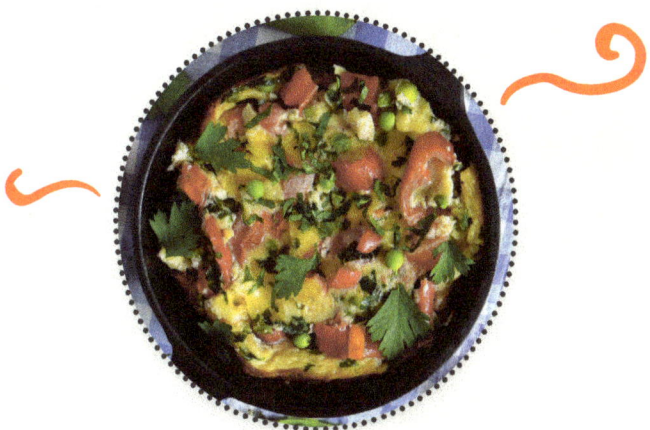

NUTRITIONAL VALUE:

Contains vitamin A, B1, B2, B3, B5, B6, B9, B12. Super high in Vitamin C, D and K. High in Protein and dietary fibre. Contains minerals and trace minerals such as Magnesium, phosphorus, potassium, calcium, zinc, iron, copper Manganese, Iodine, Sulphur, Choline, Selenium, and cancer-fighting selenium, algin, lignans, fucoidan, sulfated fucans, L-tryptophan, and iodine. This recipe includes ingredients with antioxidants and some levels of quercetin which can help with inflammation, asthma, gout, viral infections, chronic fatigue syndrome (CFS), preventing cancer, and for treating chronic infections of the prostate.

We have included ingredients that have been shown to improve liver function and boost immunity, and used as part of treatment for Prostate and Breast cancer, bowel cancer, stomach cancer and skin cancer cells. Ingredients to help soothe the nervous system, help to relieve bloating and boost digestion, regulate sugar levels and improve eye health.

Sweet Potato Wedges with Sour Cream and Chive Dip

You will need: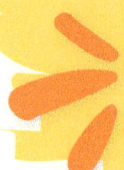

WEDGES

2 large sweet potatoes

3 tbsp Coconut oil, olive oil or 1 tbsp home-made butter

1 tbsp powdered or grated fresh turmeric

Small handful of fresh coriander

1/2 tsp Himalayan sea salt

WEDGES

125g soaked raw cashew nuts (soak for a few hours or overnight in filtered water and drain in the morning)

125ml filtered water

1 tbsp chives

1 tsp Vitamin C powder

1/2 tsp Himalayan sea salt

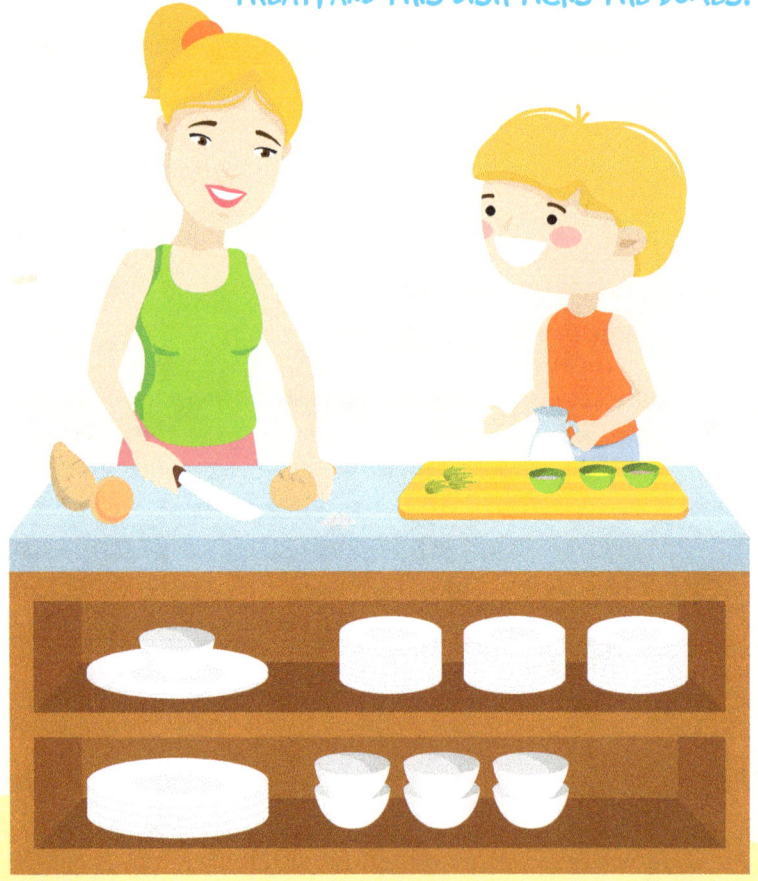

THERE IS ALWAYS A DELICIOUS HEALTHY ALTERNATIVE THAT STILL FEELS LIKE A TREAT, AND THIS DISH TICKS THE BOXES.

TO MAKE (WEDGES):

1. Wash well and soak in filtered water with 1 tspn bicarbonate soda for 12 minutes (this removes parasites, insecticides, pesticides etc)
2. Rinse and soak for 1-2 minutes in filtered water
3. Chop into wedges and boil for approx 8-10 minutes (until starts to lose hardness)
4. Drain and add oil/butter, herbs and sea salt
5. Mix gently to cover all of the wedges and turn into a glass oven dish
6. Cook for 30-40 minutes or until slightly crisp, turning half way through

TO MAKE (SOUR CREAM AND CHIVE DIP):

1. Blend all ingredients until smooth
2. Refrigerate for at least 30 minutes as this will thicken the dip

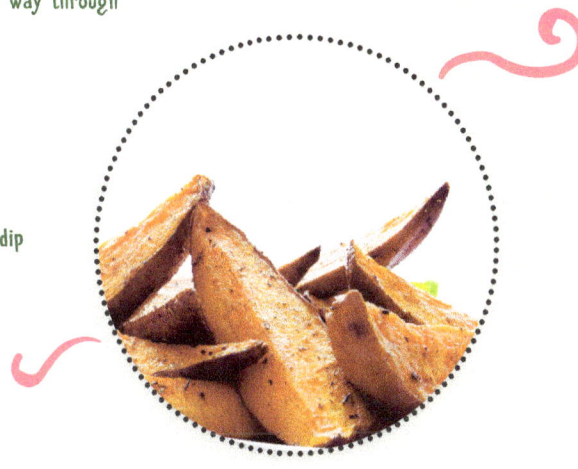

NUTRITIONAL VALUE:

Contains Vitamins A, B9, C, K and high levels of iron, plus fibre, and minerals and trace minerals such as magnesium, potassium, calcium, zinc, choline, copper, phosphorus, and manganese. An abundance of antioxidants and anti-inflammatory properties plus those that have been shown to inhibit tumours. A few science studies have shown that curcumin has anti-cancer effects. It has the best effects on breast cancer, bowel cancer, stomach cancer and skin cancer cells. At this time, there isn't enough evidence to recommend curcumin for preventing *or treating cancer, but research is ongoing. Curcumin, is a compound found in the spice turmeric.* This recipe contains high VITAMIN C and this vitamin is necessary for the growth, development and repair of all body tissues. It's involved in many body functions, including formation of collagen, absorption of iron, the immune system, wound healing, and the maintenance of cartilage, bones, and teeth.

Upside Down Mini Pizza

MAKES 2

YOU WILL NEED:

BASE:

- 400g free range turkey mince or chicken mince
- 2 tbsp Quinoa/pumpkin seed/almond/coconut flour
- 2 tbsp Olive oil
- 2 cloves Garlic
- 1 small shallot
- Small handful of chopped coriander
- 1 inch turmeric or 1 tbsn powdered
- Tomato puree or homemade pesto
- Selection of topping choices*

MAKE LUNCH FUN, FILLING AND AN ACTIVITY FOR ALL WITH A HEALTHY PIZZA BASE, AND BE CREATIVE WITH YOUR TOPPING.

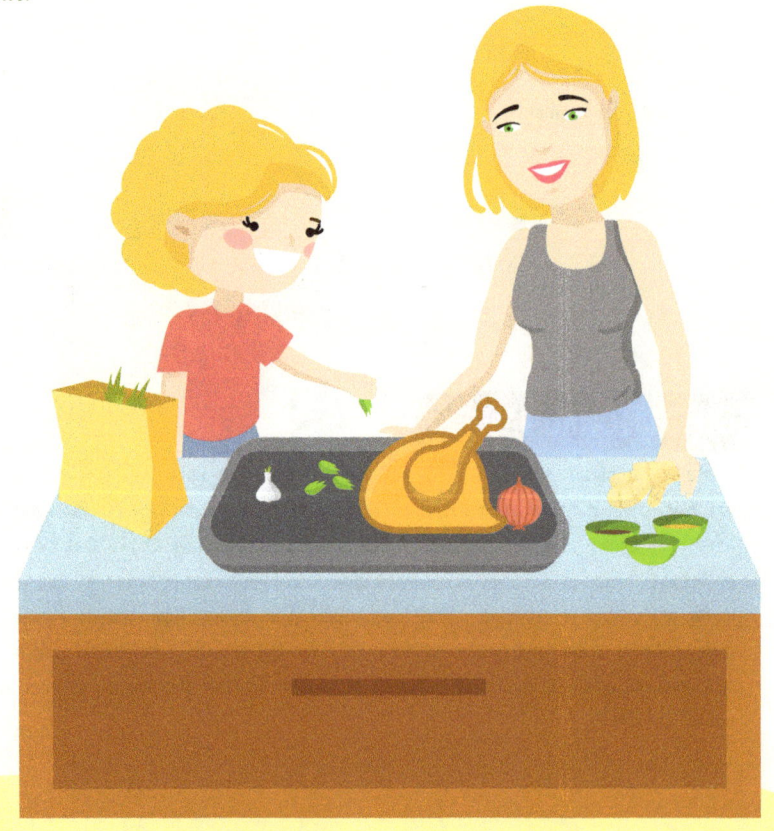

To Make:

1. Mix and mash the mince together in a glass bowl
2. Add the garlic and small shallot as well as the chopped coriander and turmeric
3. Add 2 tbsp of GF quinoa/pumpkin seed/almond/coconut flour and olive oil
4. Flatten out on an oven tray, and shape to a circle, oval or square of choice
5. Oven on 200C for 10-12 minutes
6. Remove from oven
7. Spread tomato puree or homemade *pesto (*recipe in snacks and extras section*) onto your pizza base

Topping choices:

1. Spinach, sweet peppers, olives and cashew nut cheese, sea salt and pepper
2. Shallots, pasture fed ham, peas and asparagus, Italian seasoning
3. Cashew nut cheese, tomato with fresh basil
4. Wild or wholegrain rice, tomato, pak choi, shitakii mushroom, cumin, coriander

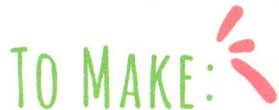

Nutritional Value:

A very rich source of protein, and B-Vitamins (B1, B2, B3, B5, B6, B9), as well as A, C, D, E, and K, along with the amino acid tryptothan essential for growth and containing anti-cancer properties. Useful minerals such as phosphorus, potassium, magnesium, zinc, calcium, copper and iron, as well as trace minerals like iodine, selenium, sulfur, choline, plus chromium-a trace mineral that enhances the ability of insulin to transport glucose from the bloodstream into cells.

This recipe will help to boost immunity, act as a powerful anti-inflammatory and digestive aid, and contains strong antimicrobial, anti-bacterial and anti-oxidants that help to fight free radicals in the body. Also a dietary source of the antioxidant lycopene, which has been linked to many health benefits, including reduced risk of heart disease and cancer. Ingredients have been included that have been shown to improve liver function, and used as part of treatment of Prostate and Breast cancer.

Bone Broth

YOU WILL NEED:

1 organic free range whole chicken

A SIMPLE AND DELICIOUS RECIPE THAT BOOSTS IMMUNITY, GUT HEALTH, SKIN HEALTH, REDUCES INFLAMMATION AND HELPS STRENGTHEN BONES AND TEETH.

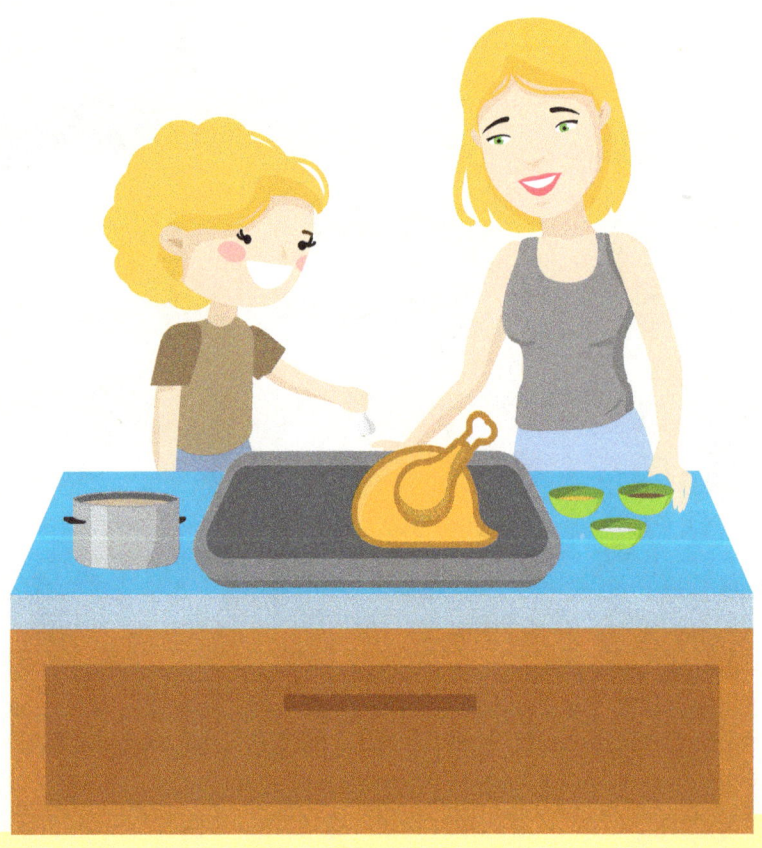

How To Make:

1. Oven cook the chicken
2. Debone and store the meat in the fridge and/or freezer for later use
3. Place the bones into a large saucepan and add enough filtered water to cover all of the bones
4. Bring to the boil and skim off any froth that is presenting on the surface
5. Simmer for up to 2-12 hours (less simmer for lower histamine, but more simmer for higher nutritional goodness)

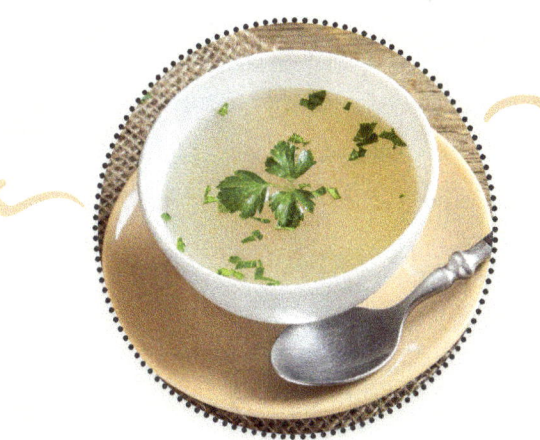

NUTRITIONAL VALUE:

Contains collagen which supports joint pain, skin health, muscle and digestive health, and amino acids like glycine and glutamine that help keep your gut working properly, which aids in digestion and keeps your immune system in check, helping to also reduce inflammation, improve hydration, and strengthen bones and teeth.

Potassium Broth

YOU WILL NEED:

8 organic red skinned potatoes
8 organic carrots
4 stalk of celery
Small handful fresh parsley
Large saucepan of filtered water

AN OLD FASHIONED MEDICAL REMEDY THAT IS FULL OF NUTRIENTS. CAN BE TAKEN ON ITS OWN OR ADDED TO OTHER MEALS AS A STOCK.

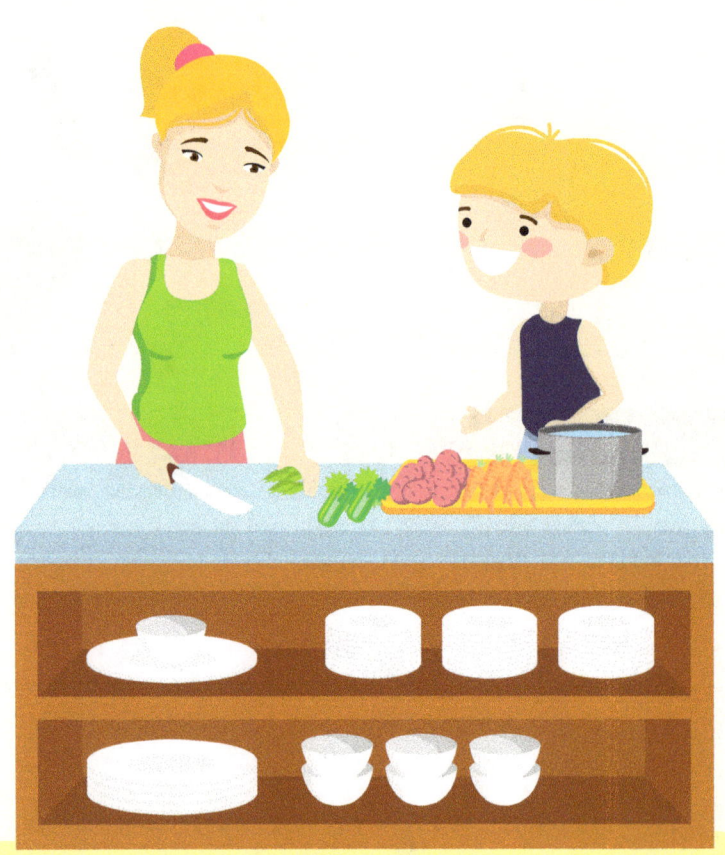

How To Make:

1. Scrub the vegetables well and peel
2. Add the peelings, parsley and celery into a bowl of filtered water with 1 tsp bicarbonate of soda, soak for 12 minutes
3. Replace with clean filtered water and soak for 2 minutes
4. Now they are clean and ready to use
5. Add the peelings and celery to the saucepan of water and bring to the boil
6. Skim away any froth that may appear on the surface
7. Once boiling bring down to a simmer for 1 hour
8. Strain and store in glass airtight containers
9. Serve warm and enjoy

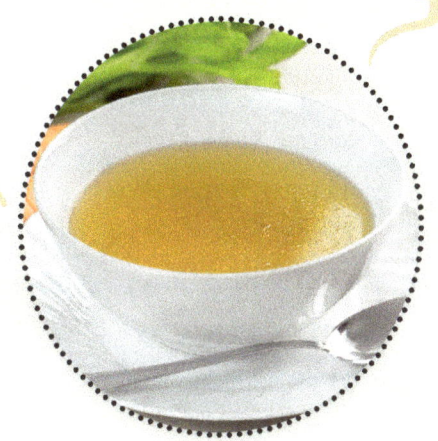

NUTRITIONAL VALUE:

A great source of hydration and immunity boost. Helps to alkalinize pH, help eliminate brain fog, improve memory, and ward off mood swings. Maintaining adequate potassium nutrition levels has also been linked to faster wound healing, diminished stress levels, lower blood pressure, and a reduction in age-related bone loss. Helps to flush system of toxins, poisons and unwanted salts and acids and give a concentrated amount of vitamins and minerals.

Creamy Vegetable Soup

SUITABLE FOR FREEZING

Ingredients:

5 Veggie Soup with Shell Pasta
A knob of butter
1 small onion, finely chopped
courgette, diced
red pepper, deseeded and diced
1 medium carrot, peeled and diced
600 ml chicken stock
2 tbsp tinned sweetcorn
1 to 2 tbsp double cream
25g shell pasta
1 tsp cornflour

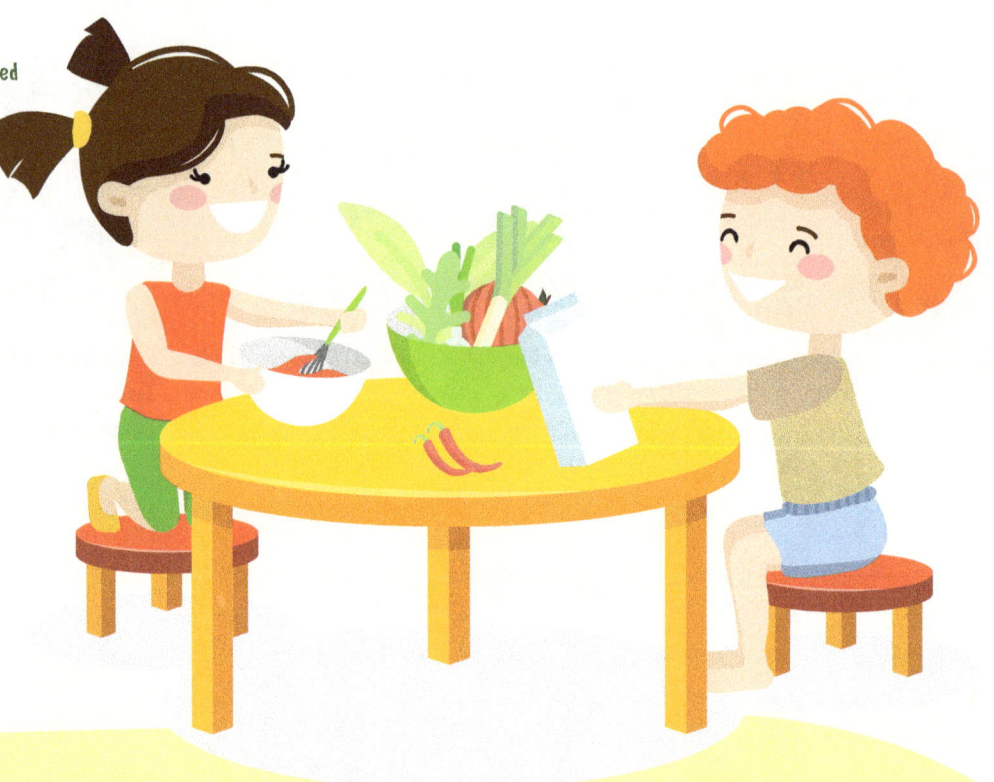

Page 60 MONSTER FIGHTING RECIPES

METHOD: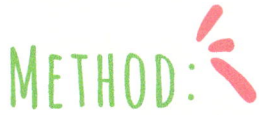

1. Melt the butter in a saucepan. Add the onion, courgette, red pepper and carrot. Fry for 5 minutes. Add the stock, then simmer for 10 minutes. Cook the pasta in boiling water according to the packet instructions and add to the soup.

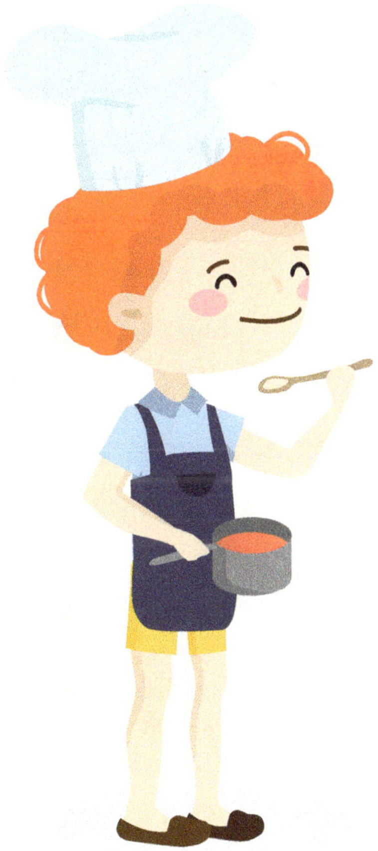

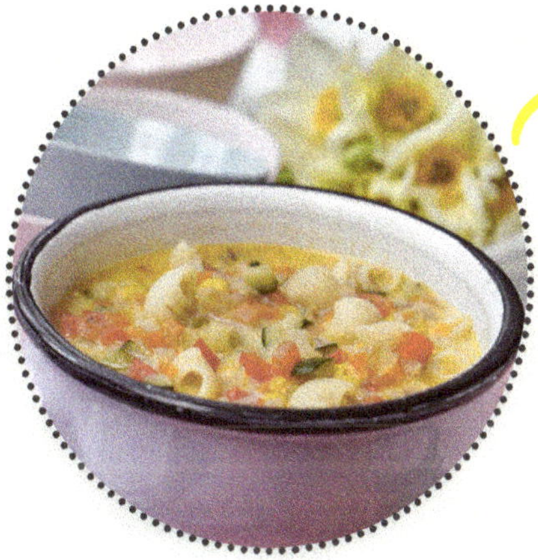

Oven Baked Chicken Nuggets

MAKES 4

Ingredients:

40g Panko breadcrumbs
40g Rice Krispies
25g finely grated parmesan
1/2 tsp paprika
2 tbsp sunflower oil
2 large chicken breasts cut into cubes
1 egg, beaten
A little plain flour

SUITABLE FOR FREEZING UNCOOKED

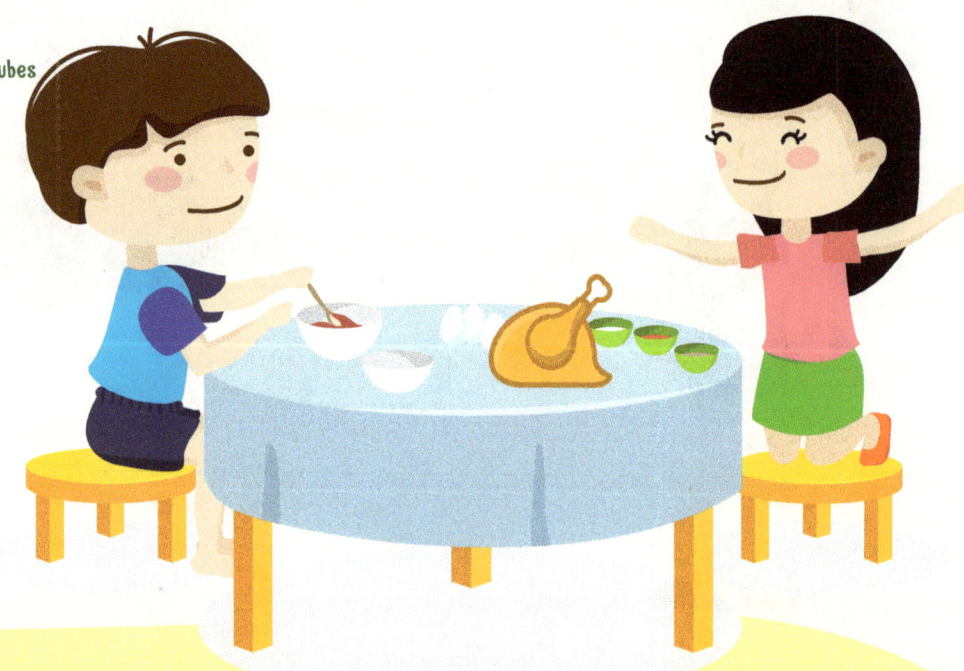

Method:

1. Preheat the oven to 200C Fan. Grease a baking sheet with oil.
2. Mea sure the Rice Krispies and Panko breadcrumbs into a plastic bag. Bash with a rolling pin until finely crushed. Add the cheese, paprika and oil and shake well.
3. Coat the chicken in flour, then dip into egg and then into the crumb mix.
4. Arrange the chicken on a baking sheet and bake in the oven for 12 to 15 minutes until golden and cooked through.

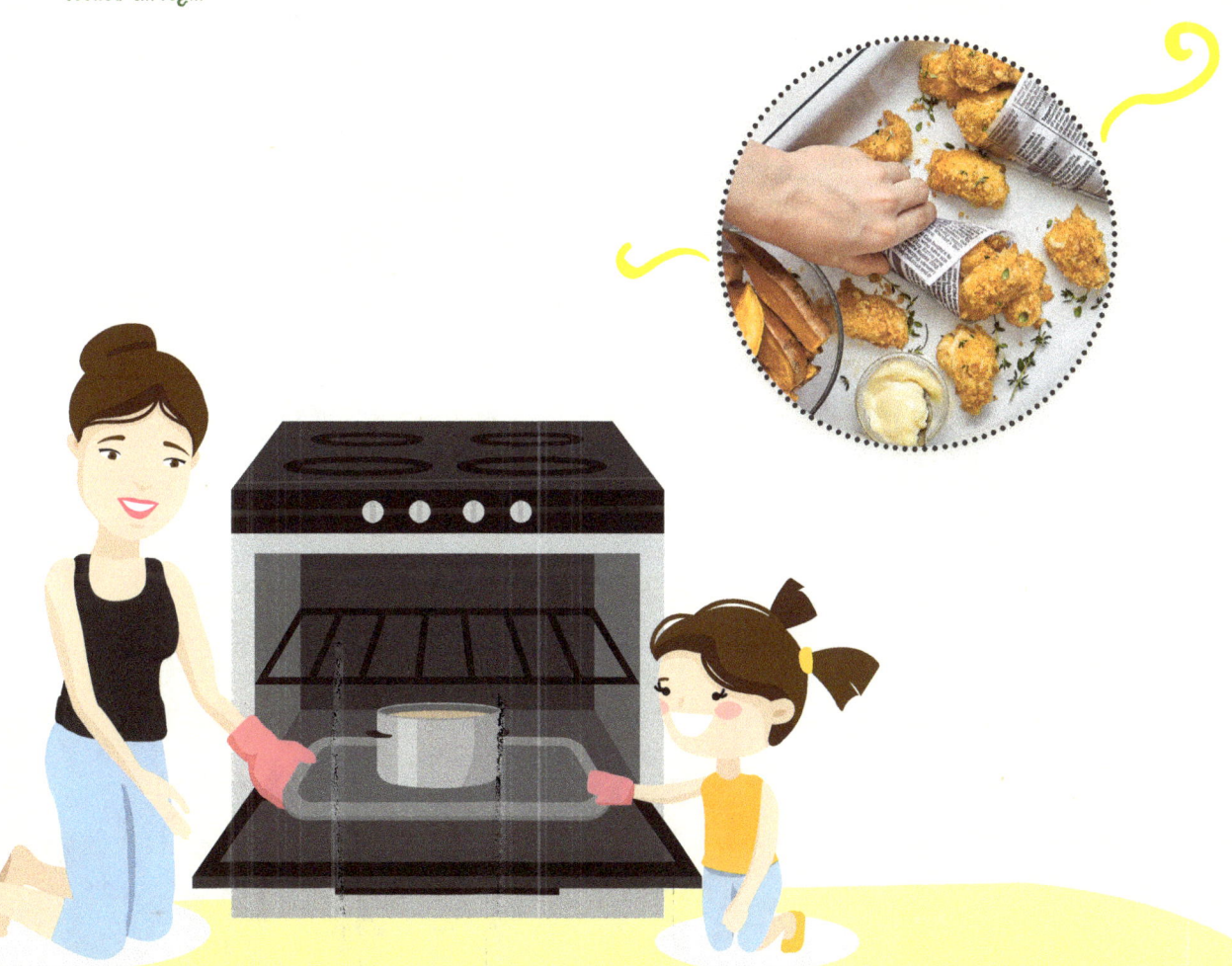

Baked Potato Mice

MAKES 4 POTATO MICE

Ingredients:

4 medium baking potatoes
A little vegetable oil
1/2 medium butternut squash
40g butter
40g parmesan, grated
1/2 tsp Dijon mustard
40g grated cheese

A FUN AND INVENTIVE WAY OF LIVENING UP JACKET POTATOES. SIMPLY MORPH THEM INTO MICE BY LETTING THE KIDS DECORATE THEM.

Decoration:

4 small cherry tomatoes
Chives
4 radishes
8 raisins
4 spring onions

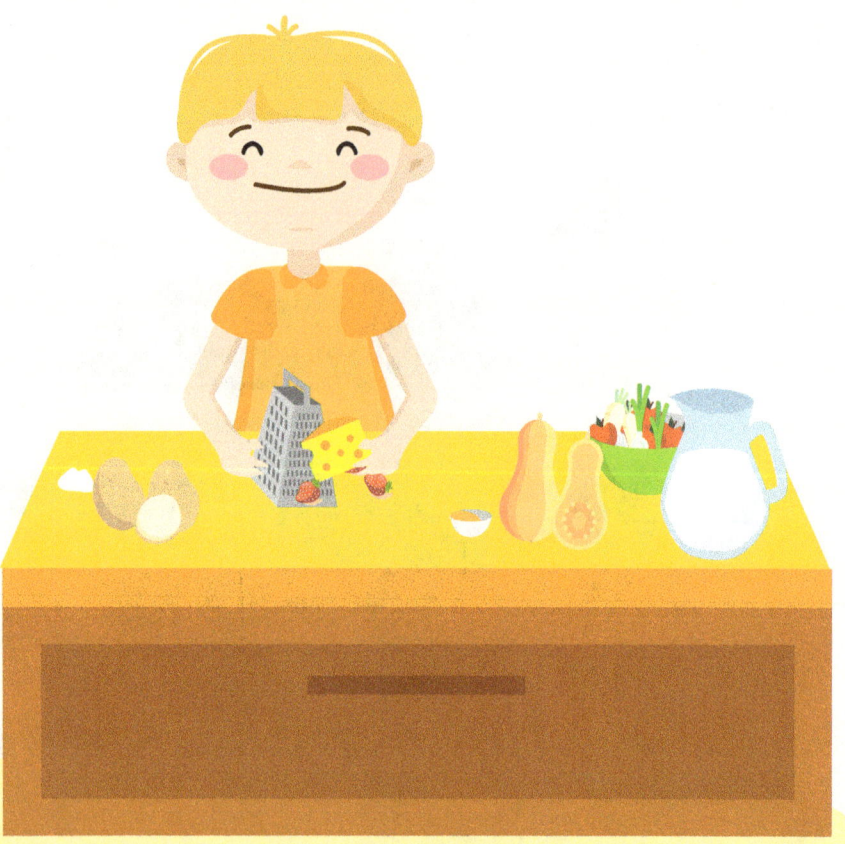

Method: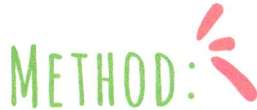

1. Prick the potatoes in several places. Place on a baking tray and brush all over with the oil. Bake in an oven preheated to 190C for 1 to 1 1/4 hours or until they feel soft when pressed.
2. Cut a medium butternut squash in half, scoop out the seeds and brush with a knob of melted butter and bake in the oven for about 40 minutes or until tender.
3. When cool enough to handle, cut the tops off the baked potatoes and scoop out the flesh. Scoop out the flesh of the cooked butternut squash and mash together with the baked potato flesh, mustard, parmesan, milk and butter. Season with a little salt and pepper. Put the mixture back into the potato shells, cover with the grated Cheddar and cook under a preheated grill for a few minutes until golden.
4. Fix a small cherry tomato into each of the potatoes using a cocktail stick for the noses. Add some short lengths of chives for the whiskers – you can tuck these behind the tomato. Decorate with halved radishes for the ears, raisins for the eyes and spring onion for the tails. You need to buy a few bunches of spring onions as you need to find the ones with the pointed ends.

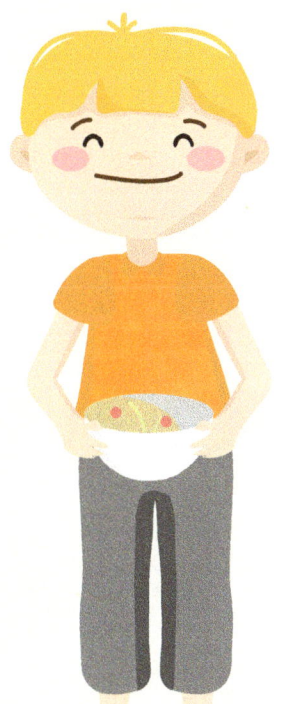
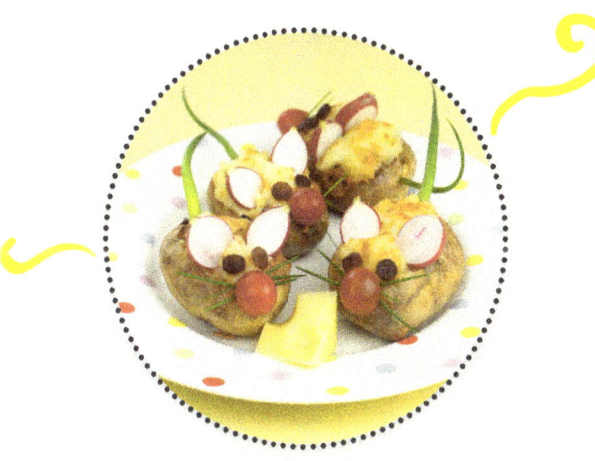

Chicken with Tomatoes and Orzo

MAKES 4 PORTIONS

INGREDIENTS:

THIS RECIPE IS FROM MY BABY LED WEANING RECIPE BOOK

3 tbsp olive oil

1 red onion, diced

1 sweet red pepper, finely diced

75g diced courgette

50g diced carrot

2 cloves garlic, crushed

1 tsp Spanish sweet smoked paprika

1 tsp good quality balsamic vinegar

125g orzo pasta

450 ml hot chicken stock

250 ml passata

1 tsp fresh or dried thyme, chopped

10 cherry tomatoes, quartered

2 ready cooked chicken breasts cut into strips

A handful of fresh basil leaves, chopped

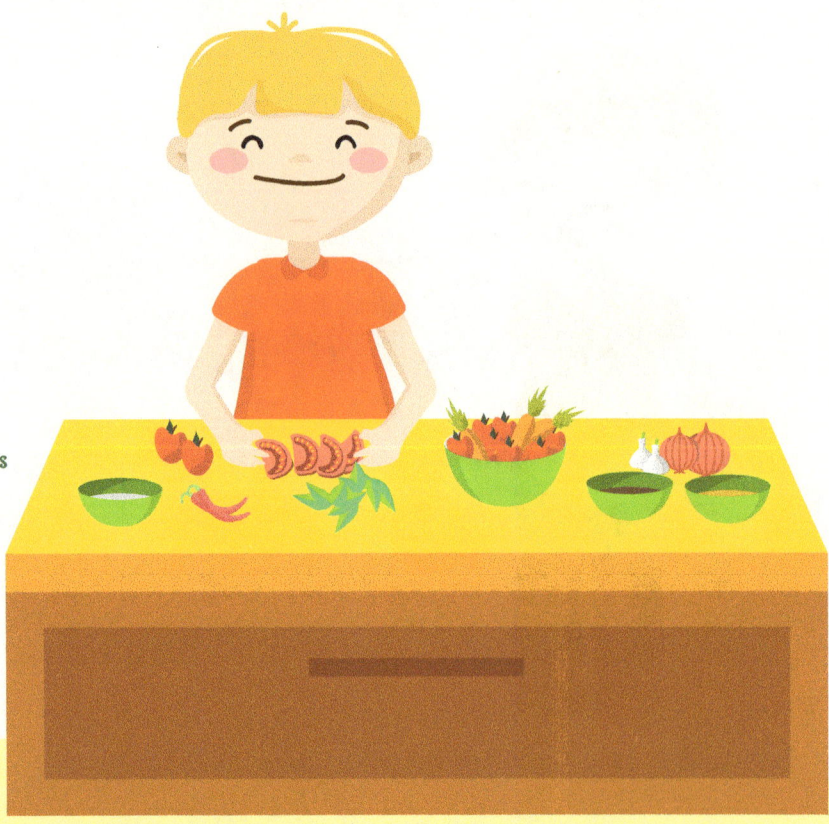

Method: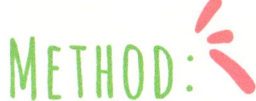

1. Heat 1 tbsp of oil in a deep frying pan. Add the onion, red pepper, courgette and carrot and fry for 3 to 4 minutes.

2. Add the garlic and sweet smoked paprika and fry for 30 seconds, then add the balsamic vinegar and orzo. Stir to coat the pasta in the mixture, then add the stock, passata and thyme. Bring to the boil, cover and simmer until cooked through for about 15 to 20 minutes or until the pasta is cooked and most of the liquid has been absorbed. Add the thyme and cherry tomatoes and stir until the tomatoes have softened slightly.

3. Add the cooked chicken strips and heat through.

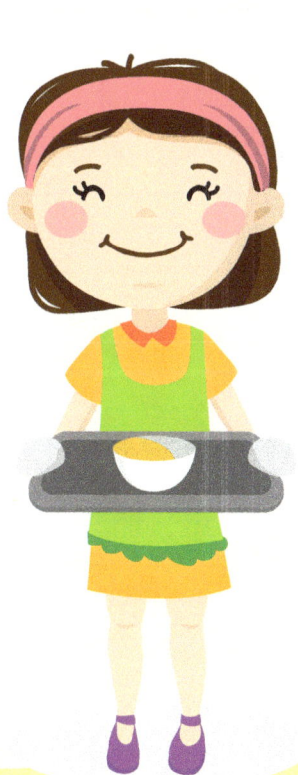

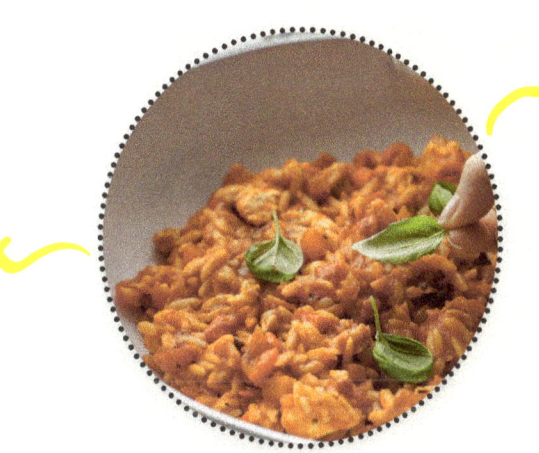

Steak and Egg on Pumpkin 'Toast'

SERVES 4

DESCRIPTION:

This fun version of steak and eggs on toast – in which the toast is replaced with a slice of roast pumpkin – makes for the most indulgent breakfast, lunch or dinner. As this dish really only takes 15-20 minutes from start to finish, it is something I throw together regularly for my family. The fact that it combines yummy fats and animal proteins with some delicious veg is perfect.

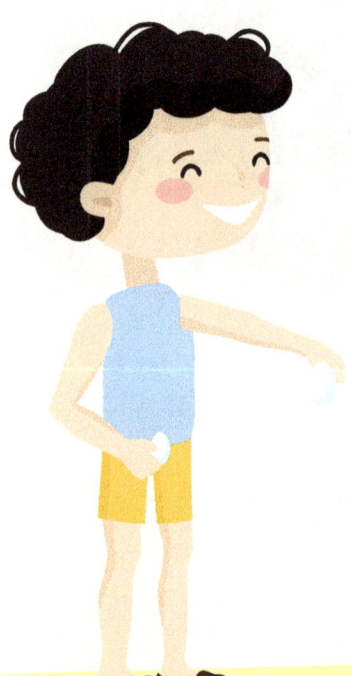

INGREDIENTS:

Butternut pumpkin 500 g, seedless part only

Minute steaks 4 x 150 g, at room temperature

Eggs 4

Melted coconut oil or good-quality animal fat 80 ml (1/3 cup)

Sea salt and freshly ground black pepper

South American dressing 80 ml (1/3 cup) (see the next recipe)

Method: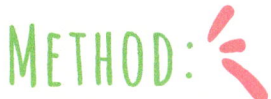

1. Preheat the oven to 220°C (200°C fan-forced). Line a baking tray with baking paper.
2. Cut the pumpkin into four slices about 2 cm thick, then rub the cut sides with 1 tablespoon of the coconut oil or fat and season with salt and pepper. Place the pumpkin on the prepared tray in a single layer and roast for 15 minutes, then flip and roast for a further 15 minutes, or until the pumpkin is cooked through and golden. Set aside to cool slightly.
3. Meanwhile, heat 2 tablespoons of the coconut oil or fat in a large frying pan over high heat. Season the steaks with salt and pepper. Cook on one side for 2 minutes, then flip and cook the other side for 1-2 minutes (or cook to your liking). Transfer to a plate and allow to rest for 2 minutes, keeping warm.
4. Wipe the pan clean, place over medium heat and add the remaining 1 tablespoon of coconut oil or fat. Crack in the eggs and cook for 2 and half minutes, or until the egg whites are set (or cook to your liking). Season with salt and pepper.
5. Place the pumpkin toast on serving plates, top with a minute steak and a fried egg. Spoon over the dressing and serve.

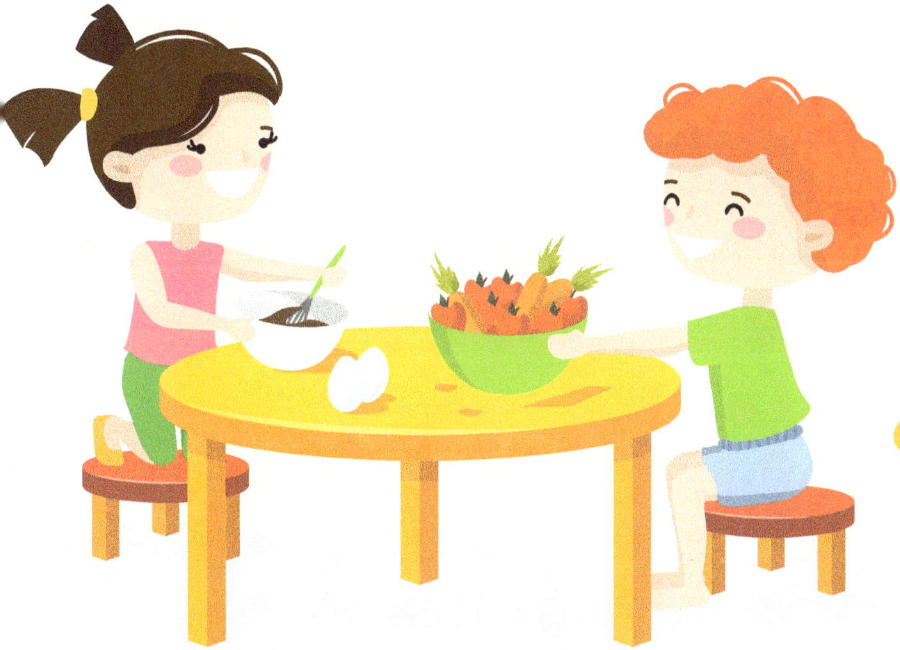

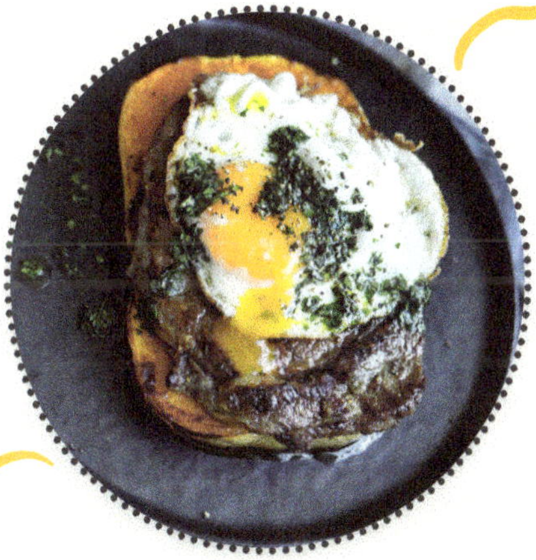

Page 70 MONSTER FIGHTING Recipes

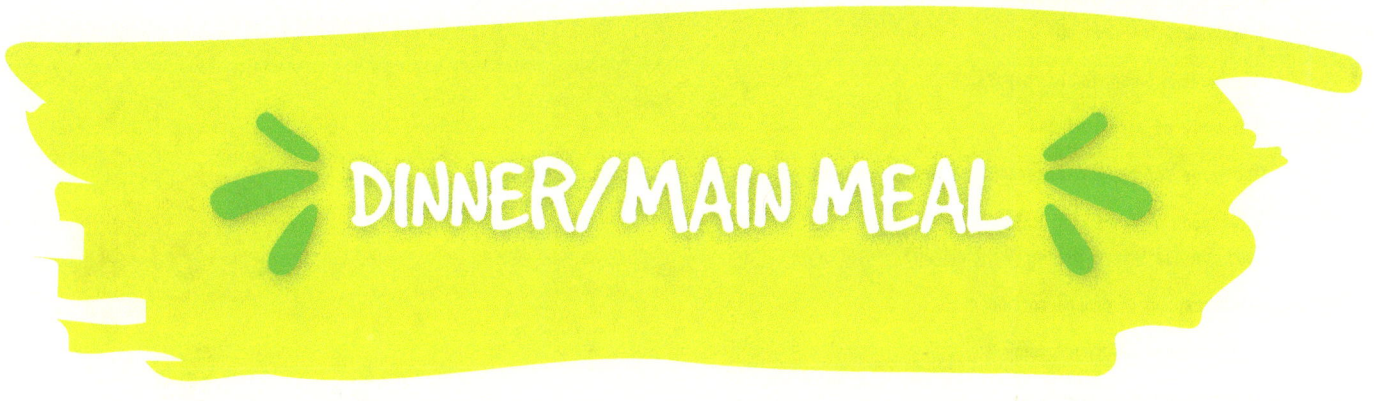

Vegan Black Bean and Lentil Chili with nacho Chips

Serves: 2 adults | Prep: 20 mins | Cooking time: 50 mins

Ingredients:

For the chili:

1 tablespoon of olive oil

One medium onion, finely chopped

One clove of garlic, minced

One large red pepper, deseeded and finely chopped

1 teaspoon of dried chili flakes
(you can use less if making for children)

1/2 teaspoon of ground coriander

1/2 teaspoon of ground cumin

2 cardamom pods, crushed

150g of red lentils

One 400g can chopped tomatoes

350ml of water

One 400g can black beans

2 tablespoons tomato ketchup

2 tablespoons of tomato purée

2 teaspoons of cocoa powder

For the nacho's:

2 tortilla wraps

Spray oil

Paprika

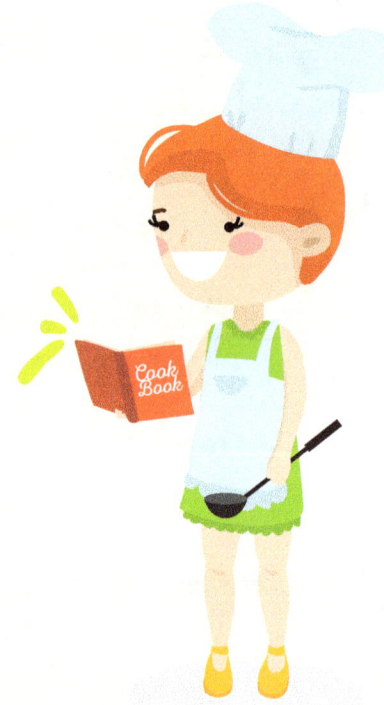

Method:

1. Prepare the vegetables as described
2. Pre-heat the oven to 160°
3. In a large pan heat the oil and fry the onion garlic and peppers until everything is soft.
4. Add the chili, coriander, cumin and cardamom pods, keep stirring being careful not to let the spices to burn.
5. Add the lentils and continue to stir for 1 minute till the spices evenly coat the lentils.
6. Add the chopped tomatoes, water, kidney beans, ketchup, tomato paste and cocoa and bring the mixture to the boil.
7. Simmer gently covered, for about 40 minutes stirring frequently, add more water if the chili looks dry
8. While the chili is simmering prepare your nachos by cutting each of the flour tortillas into eight equal sections, like a pizza.
9. Cover both sides of each nacho chip with spray oil and place on a baking tray
10. Sprinkle with paprika and bake in the preheated oven for 10-15 minutes till crisp.

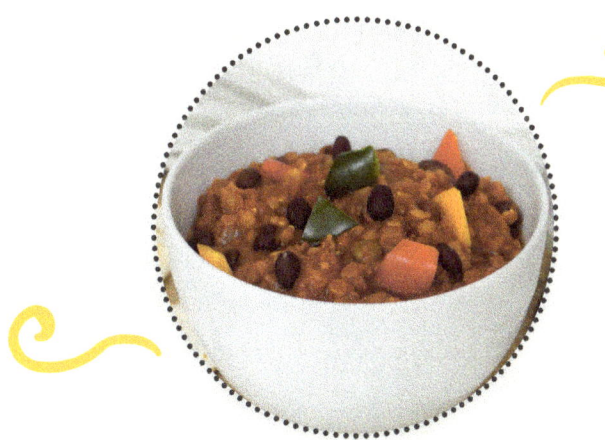

Lemon and Garlic Chicken

SERVES 4

DESCRIPTION:

This classic French dish of roast chicken with lemon, shallots and garlic is, in my mind, a perfect meal. The combination of the acidity from the lemon, mixed with the garlicky chicken juices and roast shallots really is sensational. Plus the whole thing is made in one dish!

INGREDIENTS:

Chicken 1 x 1.8 kg

Garlic bulbs 2, halved horizontality or cloves separated

Lemon 1, sliced, plus extra, cut into wedges, to serve

French shallots 8, peeled

Chicken bone broth 400 ml

Coconut oil or good-quality animal fat 3 tablespoons, melted (see note)

Sea salt and freshly ground black pepper

Flat-leaf parsley leaves finely chopped, to serve (optional)

Method:

1. Preheat the oven to 200°C (180°C fan-forced).
2. Rinse the chicken inside and out, pat dry with paper towel, then rub on the coconut oil or fat and season generously inside and out with salt and pepper. Tie the legs up with kitchen string.
3. Place the chicken in a casserole dish, scatter around the garlic, lemon slices and shallots and pour in the broth. Roast, basting occasionally with the juices in the dish, for 40 minutes. Reduce the temperature to 170°C (150°C fan-forced) and roast for a further 30–45 minutes until the chicken is golden and the juices run clear when the thigh is pierced with a skewer. Allow the chicken to rest for 10 minutes before sprinkling on the parsley, if using, and serving with the lemon wedges.

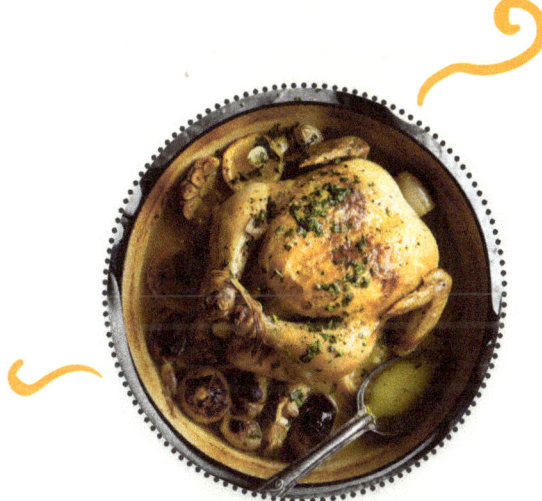

Note:

I use either coconut oil or good-quality animal fats for cooking as they have high smoke points (meaning they do not oxidise at high temperatures). Some of my favourite animal fats to use are lard (pork fat), tallow (rendered beef fat), rendered chicken fat and duck fat. These may be hard to find – ask at your local butcher or meat supplier, look online for meat suppliers who sell them or make your own when making bone broths.

Pan-Fried Snapper with Broccomole

SERVES 4

DESCRIPTION:

Holy broccomole! Broccomole is basically guacamole with some raw or cooked broccoli folded through it, which makes for an awesome accompaniment to so many things . . . eggs – poached, fried or boiled – grilled, steamed, poached or roasted meats and seafood, seed crackers, raw fish wrapped in nori, paleo nachos . . . the list goes on. Here, I demonstrate how to get a dish on the table from start to finish in under 10 minutes. Mind you, I get the girls to make the broccomole for me, so all I have to do is cook the fish and add some kraut.

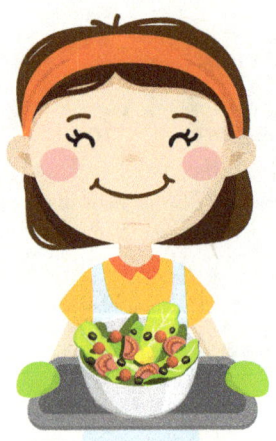

INGREDIENTS:

4 x 160 g snapper fillets, skin on or off, pin-boned

Sea salt and freshly ground black pepper

1 teaspoon lemon thyme leaves, chopped

2 tablespoons coconut oil

100 g sauerkraut

1 large handful of watercress sprigs 4 lemon wedges, to serve

Method: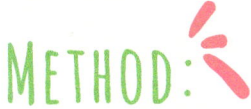

1. Season the snapper fillets with salt and pepper and sprinkle over the thyme.

2. Heat the coconut oil in a large heavy-based frying pan over high heat. Fry the fish, skin-side down and in batches if necessary, for 2 1/2–3 minutes, or until crispy. Flip over and cook for 2 minutes, or until the fish is just cooked through. Rest for 2 minutes.

3. To make the broccomole, bring a saucepan of salted water to the boil. Add the broccoli and cook for 3 minutes, or until just tender. Drain, then plunge the broccoli into ice-cold water to stop the cooking process. When the broccoli is completely cold, drain again, shake off any excess water and chop into small pieces. Place the avocado, onion, garlic, lime juice, chilli flakes (if using), olive oil, coriander and broccoli in a serving bowl and mix well. Season with salt and pepper.

4. To serve, divide the fish among four plates. Add the broccomole, sauerkraut and watercress, and drizzle with a little extra olive oil. Serve with the lemon wedges.

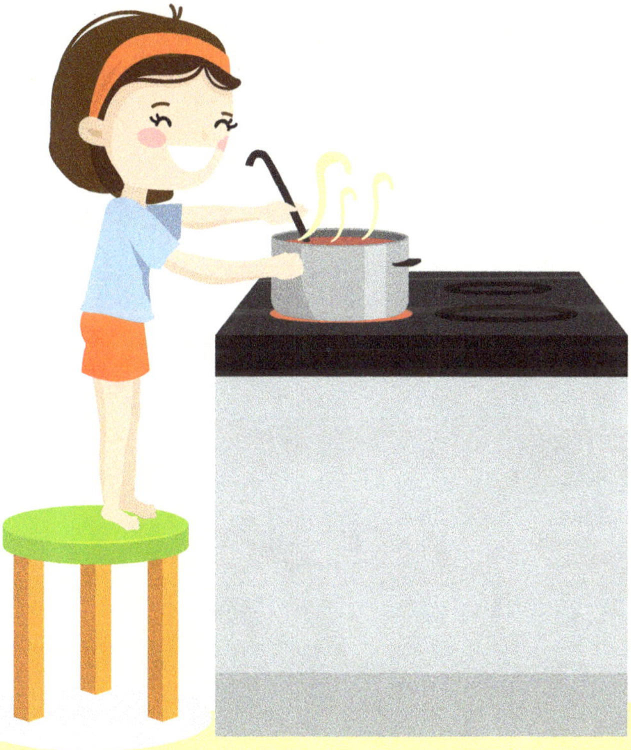

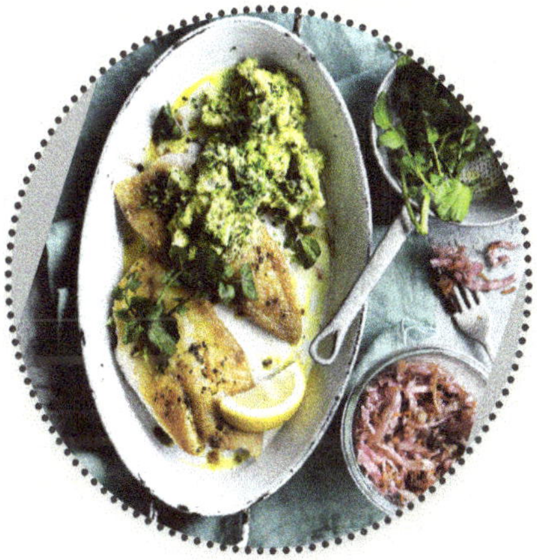

Sweet Potato Crab Cakes

PREPARATION 10 MINUTES | COOKING 35 MINUTES (PLUS 30 MINUTES CHILLING) | SERVES 4

Ingredients:

FOR THE CHILI:

Sweet potato (450g), peeled and cut into chunks

1 spring onion, chopped

Half a small red onion, finely chopped

Salt and black pepper

Dried thyme (a quarter of a teaspoon)

Fresh parsley (1 tablespoon), chopped

Half a scotch bonnet chilli pepper, deseeded and finely diced (optional)

Mayonnaise (1 tablespoon)

1 tin of crabmeat (120g), drained

Breadcrumbs (120g), natural or golden

Vegetable oil (1 tablespoon)

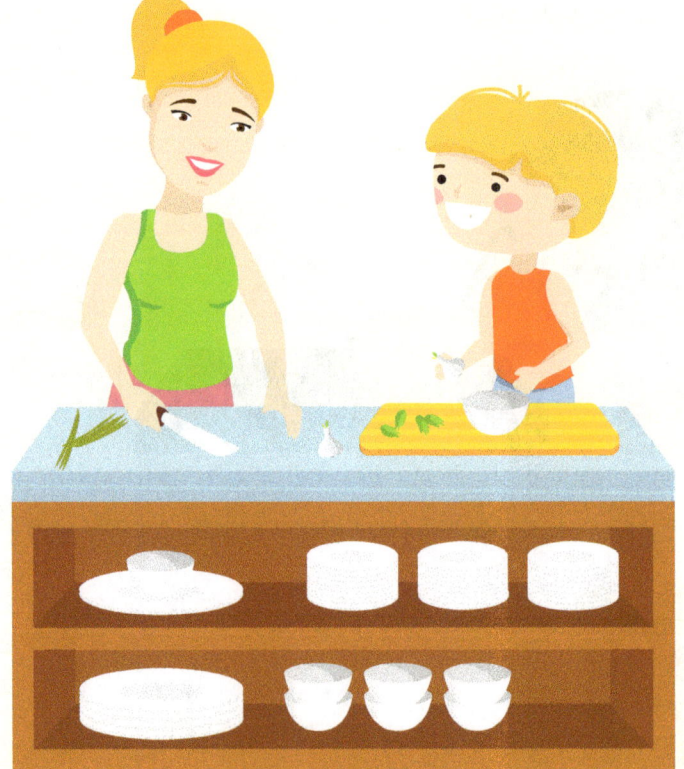

Method:

1. Cook the sweet potato in boiling water until tender. Drain it and mash it in a deep bowl.
2. When the sweet potato is cool, add all the ingredients except the crabmeat, breadcrumbs and vegetable oil. Mix well.
3. Squeeze the water from the crabmeat and fold into the mixture. Chill in the fridge for about 20 minutes.
4. Roll the mixture into balls (about the size of a golf ball). Then roll the balls in the breadcrumbs, pressing down gently so the crumbs stick. Put them in the fridge for 10 minutes to firm up.
5. In a wide pan, heat the vegetable oil over a medium heat. Press down on each crab cake ball to make a patty. Fry them on each side until golden brown, then drain them on kitchen paper to absorb the extra oil.

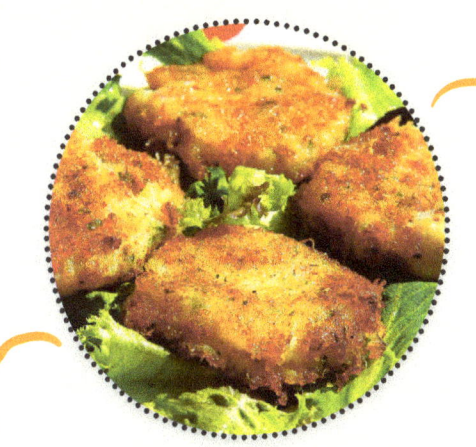

WARNING

Scotch bonnets are hot! If you have a sore mouth, leave it out. If you like less heat, use a bird's eye chilli instead.

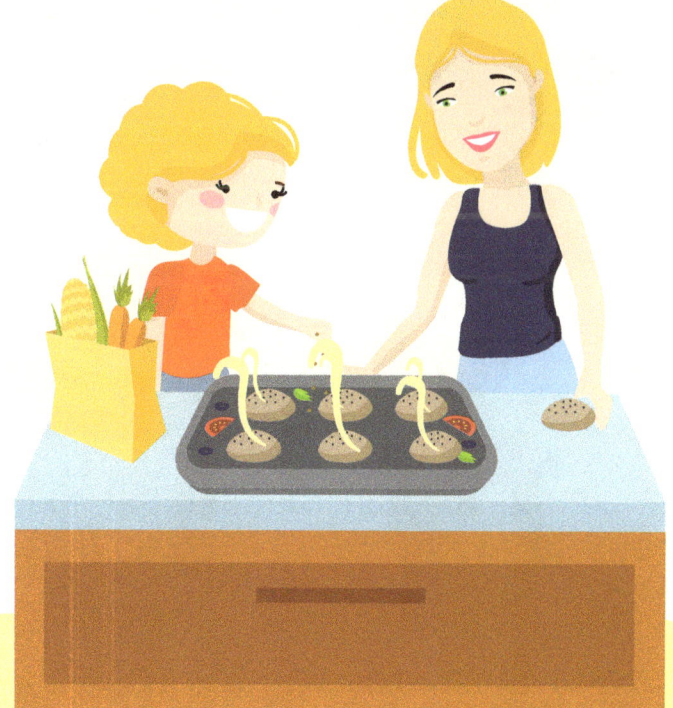

chicken and white bean salad

PREPARATION 10 MINUTES | SERVES 2

INGREDIENTS:

1 tin of haricot beans (400g), rinsed and drained

Olive oil (3 tablespoons)

Wholegrain mustard (1 tablespoon)

Zest and juice of a lemon

Rocket leaves (70g)

2 cooked chicken breasts, sliced

8 cherry tomatoes, quartered

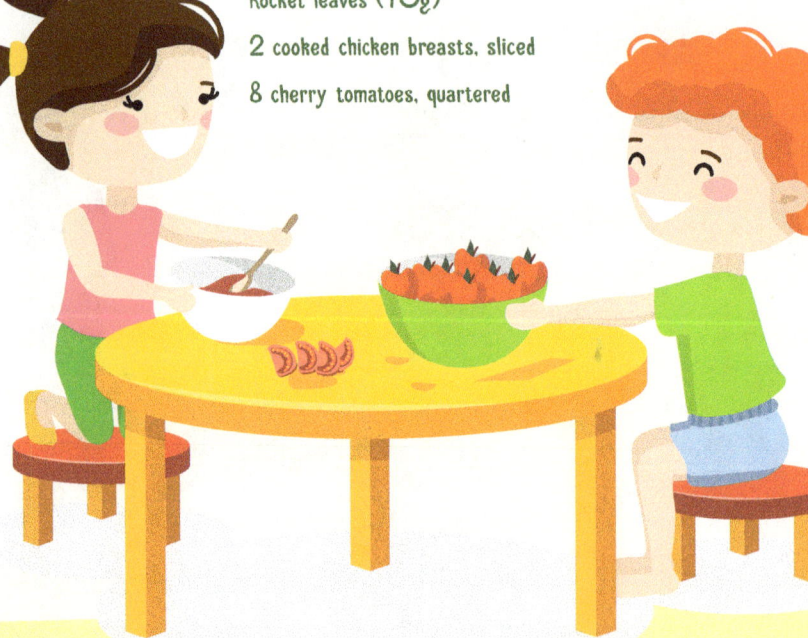

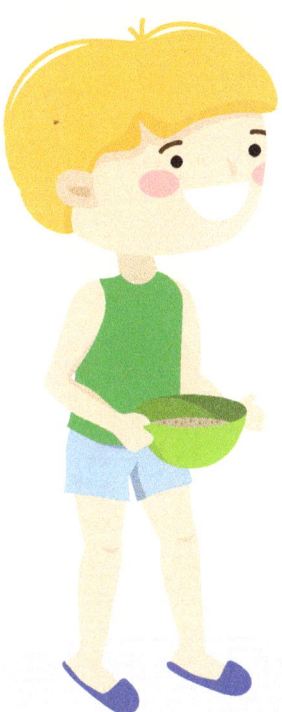

Method:

1. Whisk the oil with the mustard and lemon zest and juice.
2. Drizzle half of the dressing over the beans in a bowl. Gently toss to coat.
3. Divide the rocket between two serving dishes and then scatter with the beans.
4. 4 Add the chicken and tomatoes and then drizzle over the remaining dressing.
5. Finish with a pinch of salt and black pepper, then serve.

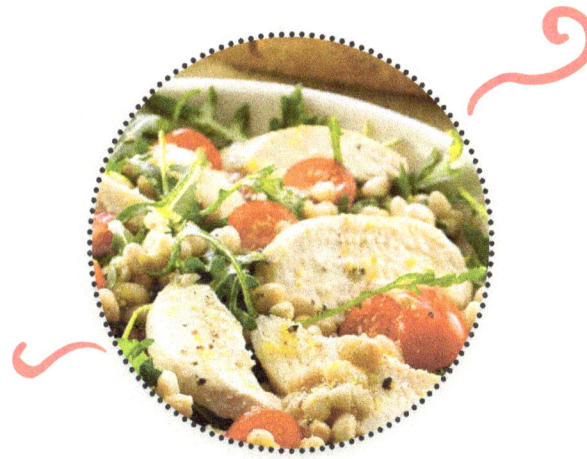

Cod Viennoise

PREPARATION 20 MINUTES | COOKING 40 MINUTES | SERVES 4

Ingredients: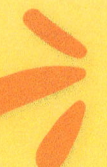

- 2 hard-boiled eggs, shells removed
- White breadcrumbs (85g)
- 4 cod steaks (140g each)
- Salt and black pepper
- Flour (40g)
- 1 egg, beaten
- Olive oil (1 tablespoon)
- Butter (75g)
- Lemon juice (1 tablespoon)
- Capers (2 tablespoons)
- 4 anchovies, chopped
- Fresh parsley (1 tablespoon), chopped

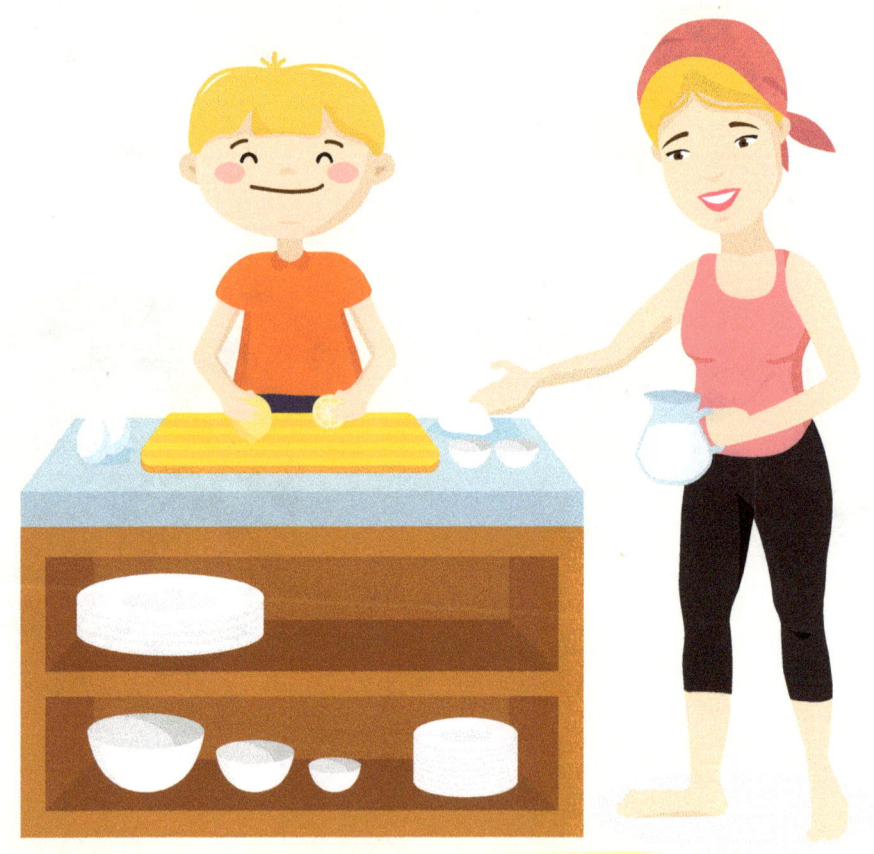

Method:

1. Preheat the oven to 180°C/160°C fan/gas mark 4.
2. Push the hard-boiled eggs through a sieve into a bowl, using your thumbs or a spoon. Mix with the breadcrumbs.
3. Remove the bones and skin from the cod steaks. Pat the steaks dry with kitchen paper.
4. Add a pinch of salt and pepper to the flour. Use this flour mix to coat the cod steaks.
5. Dip the steaks in the beaten egg, making sure they are covered on all sides. Then dip them into the breadcrumb mix, making sure the coating sticks to the fish.
6. Heat the oil with 25g of butter in a frying pan. Fry the cod steaks until they are golden brown. Then turn them over, place in an ovenproof dish and cook them in the oven for 5 to 10 minutes.
7. Meanwhile, melt the rest of the butter until it is golden-brown. Add the lemon juice, capers, anchovies and parsley.
8. Take the fish out of the oven and pour the caper butter over it before serving.

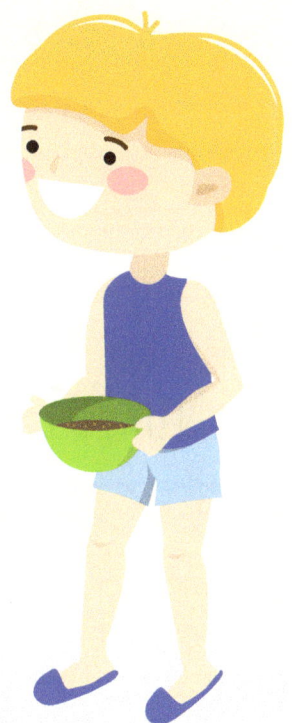

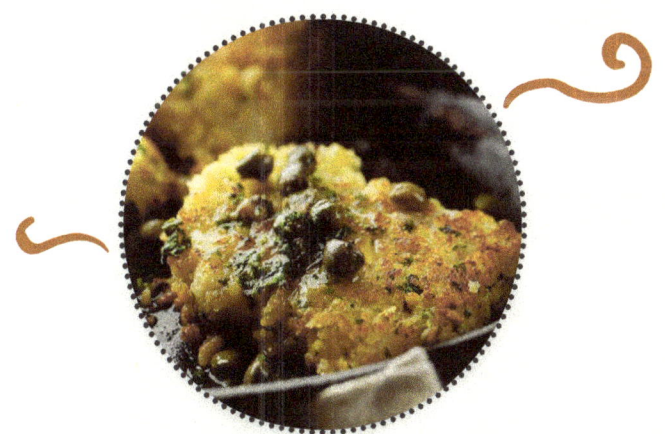

TIPS

To reduce the fat content, leave out the butter and use only a small amount of oil in a non-stick pan. A couple of sprays of a spray oil will normally be enough.

Salmon curry

PREPARATION 10 MINUTES | COOKING 20 MINUTES | SERVES 2

Ingredients:

Sunflower or vegetable oil (1 tablespoon)

1 small onion, sliced

2 garlic cloves, sliced

A quarter of a chilli pepper, deseeded and sliced

Curry powder (1 teaspoon)

1 tin of pink salmon (213g)

1 spring onion, chopped

1 tomato, chopped

Salt and black pepper

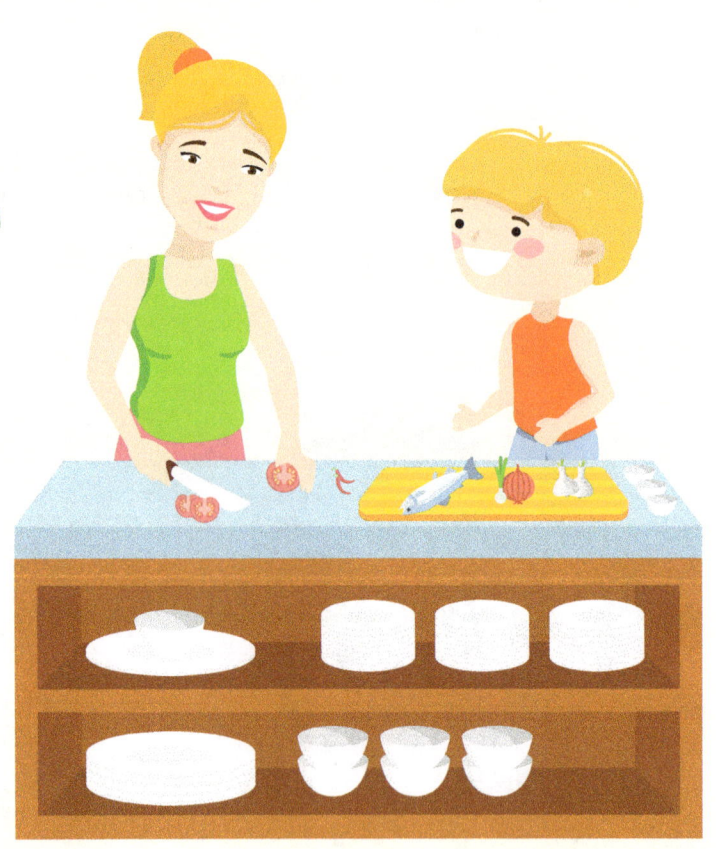

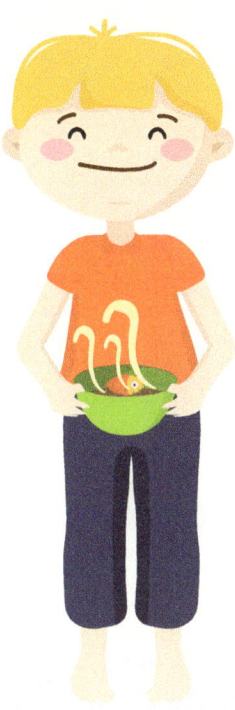

Method:

1. Heat the oil in a pan on a medium heat. Add the onion and garlic. Cook for about 2 minutes until the onions are soft.
2. Add the chilli pepper and cook for 1 minute. Then add the curry powder and cook for a further 2 minutes, stirring well.
3. Add 70ml of water and stir. Turn down the heat and cook for about 3 to 5 minutes, until all the liquid cooks off.
4. Empty the tin of salmon into a dish and remove any bones. Then empty the salmon and its liquid into the pan and break apart.
5. Stir in the spring onion, tomato, salt and black pepper. Cover and bring to the boil. Then reduce the heat to a gentle simmer for about 5 minutes, stirring occasionally but without breaking up the fish too much.
6. Serve with boiled rice or in a chapati.

TIPS

If you have a sore mouth, leave out the chilli pepper.

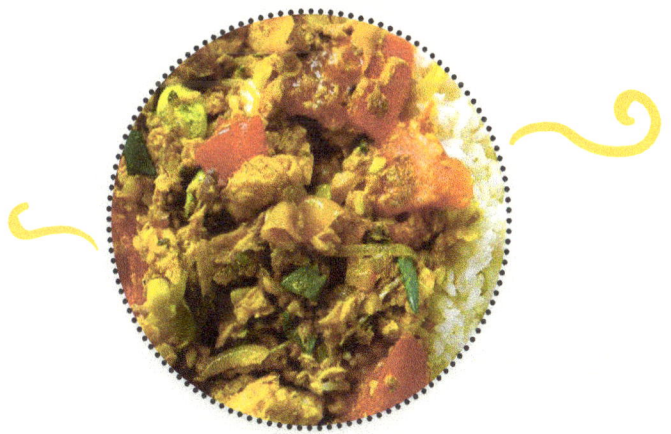

One-Pot Fish with Black Olives and Tomatoes

PREPARATION 15 MINUTES | COOKING 20 MINUTES | SERVES 4

Ingredients:

- Olive oil (2 tablespoons)
- 1 large onion, roughly chopped
- 1 tin of chopped tomatoes (400g)
- Salt and black pepper
- Black olives (175g), stones removed
- 4 boneless white fish fillets, such as cod or pollock (175g each)
- Fresh parsley (2 tablespoons), chopped
- 1 lemon, cut into wedges

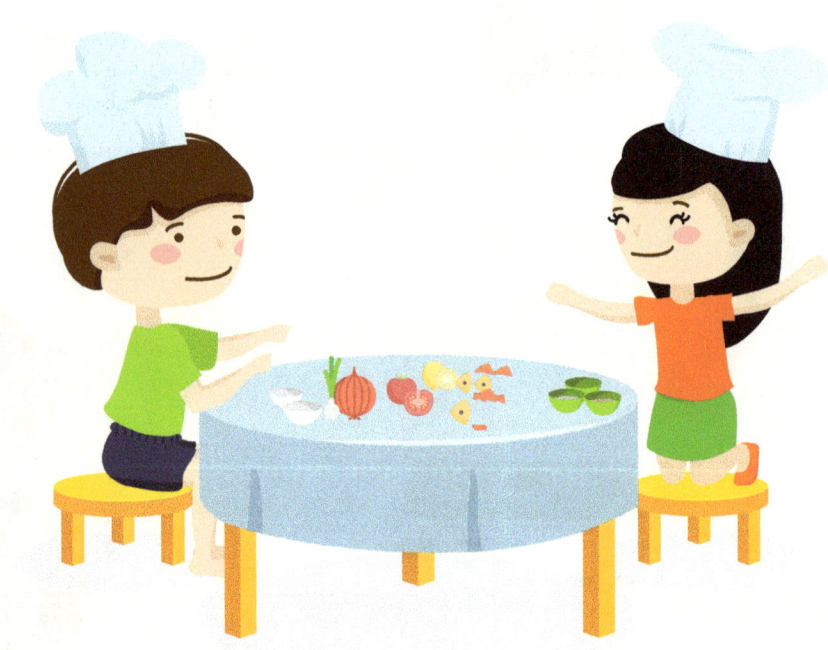

Method: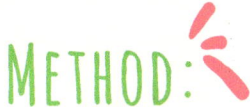

1. Preheat the oven to 200°C/180°C fan/gas mark 6.
2. Heat half the oil in an ovenproof pan. Add the onion and stir well. Leave to cook for 1 to 2 minutes, then stir again.
3. Add the tomatoes, salt and pepper. Bring to the boil, then add the olives.
4. Put the fish on top of the sauce, skin-side down. Drizzle over the rest of the oil. Bake it uncovered for 15 minutes until the fish is cooked.
5. Sprinkle with the parsley and serve straight from the pan, with lemon wedges to squeeze over the fish.

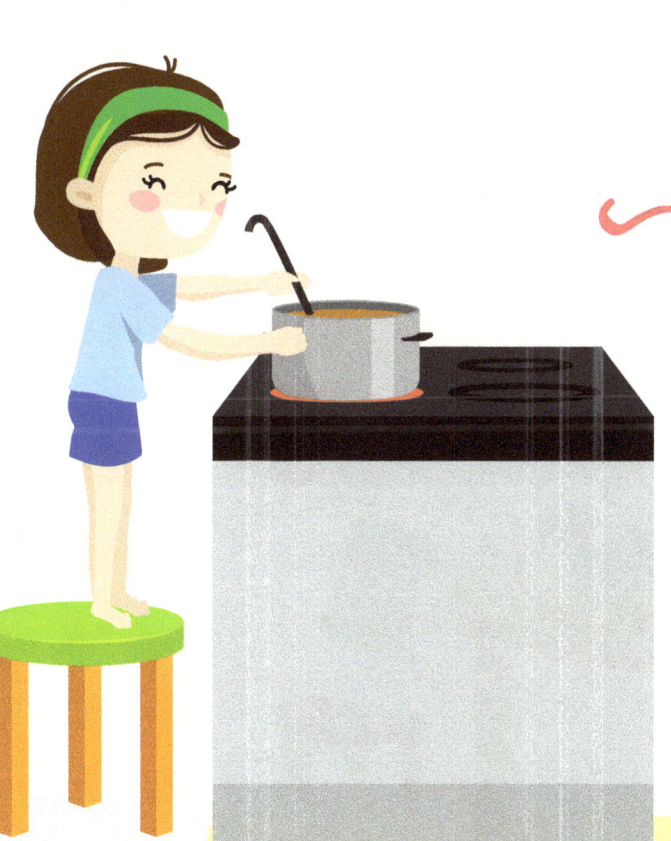

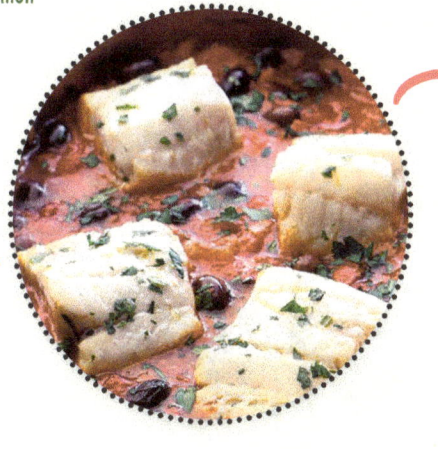

TIPS

Use a spray oil in a non-stick pan to reduce the fat content.

Tuna and Vegetable Spaghetti

PREPARATION 2 MINUTES | COOKING 15 MINUTES | SERVES 4

Ingredients:

Dry spaghetti (300g)

Frozen, mixed vegetables (400g)

1 jar of white lasagne sauce (525g)

2 tins of tuna (200g each), drained

Salt and black pepper

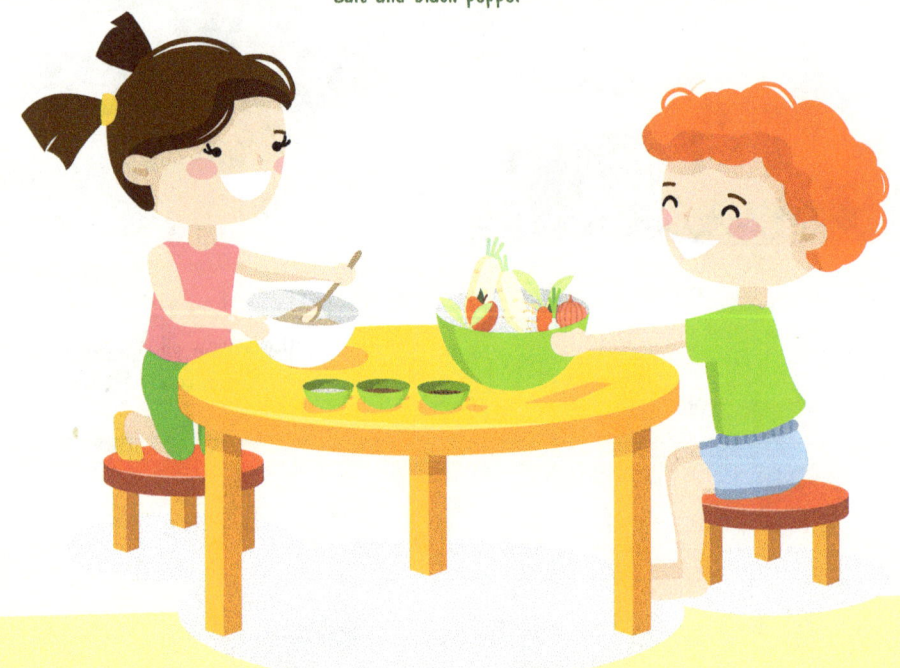

Method:

1. Boil the spaghetti in a large pan and cook according to the instructions on the packet. Add in the mixed vegetables for the last 5 minutes. Drain and leave to the side.
2. Pour the white lasagne sauce and tuna into the pan. Heat it for 1 minute.
3. Return the spaghetti and vegetables to the pan with the sauce and stir to heat it through.
4. Finish with a pinch of salt and black pepper, then serve.

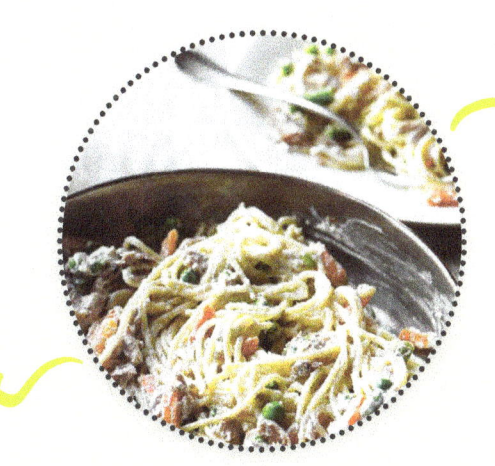

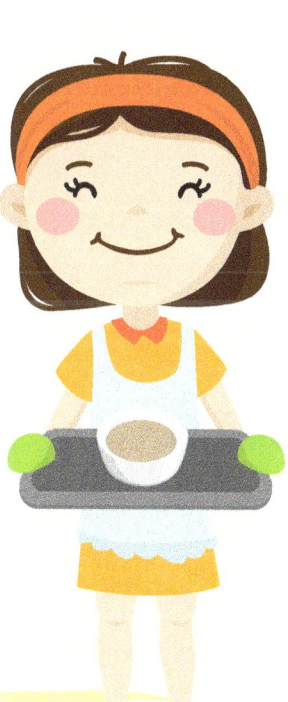

Spring onion, garlic and prawn risotto

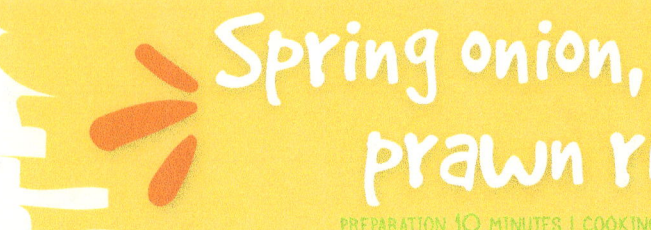

PREPARATION 10 MINUTES | COOKING 35 MINUTES | SERVES 4

Ingredients:

- Olive oil (1 tablespoon)
- 1 bunch of spring onions, chopped
- 4 garlic cloves, sliced
- Arborio rice (310g)
- Chicken stock (560ml/1 pint)
- Fish stock (560ml/1 pint)
- 20 large, cooked prawns
- Juice of half a lemon
- Parmesan cheese (1 tablespoon)
- Black pepper
- Chives (1 tablespoon), chopped

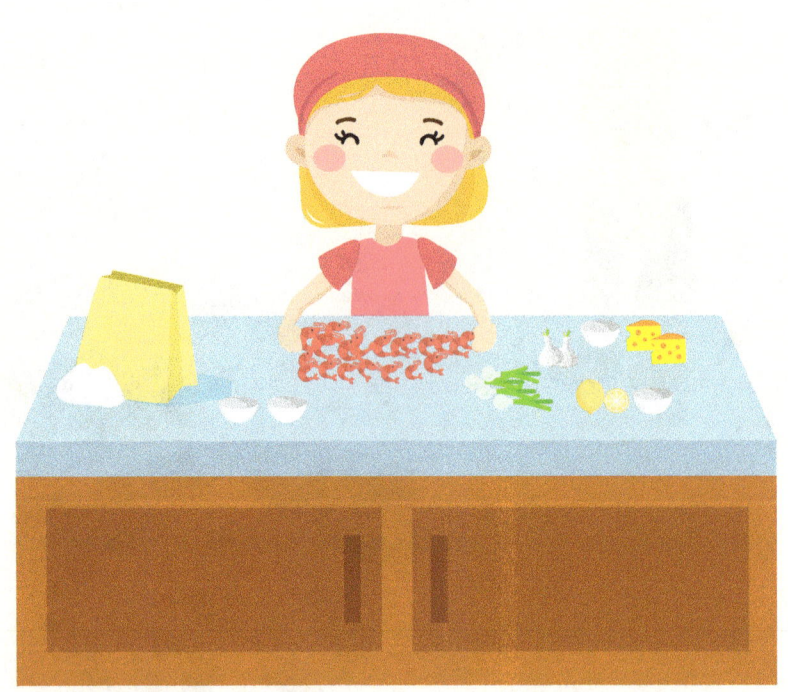

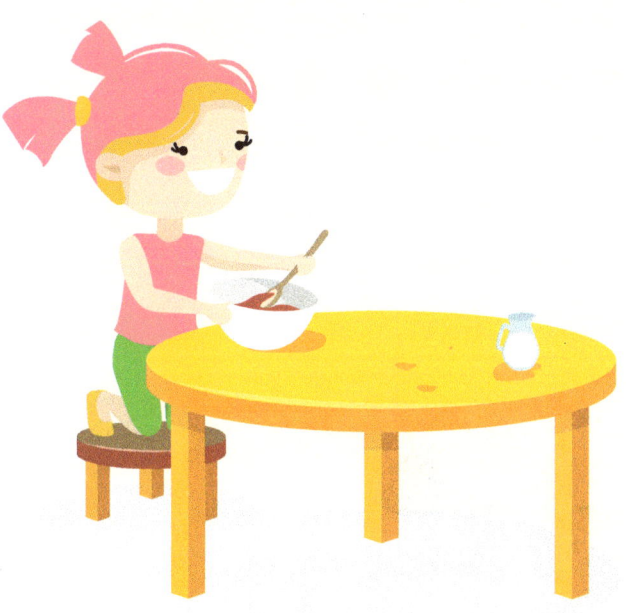

Method:

1. Heat the oil in a large frying pan.
2. Add the spring onions and garlic. Cook gently, but don't brown.
3. Add the rice and sweat until it changes colour.
4. Meanwhile, boil the stocks together in a separate pan.
5. Add about one fifth of the stock to the frying pan and bring to the boil. Leave to simmer until the liquid disappears, stirring regularly. Repeat until you have used all the stock.
6. When all the stock has been absorbed into the rice, stir in the prawns, lemon juice, parmesan and black pepper.
7. Sprinkle with the chives and serve.

TIPS

To reduce the fat content, leave out the parmesan cheese.

To increase the calories, add some cream and more cheese.

If you have problems chewing, use smaller prawns.

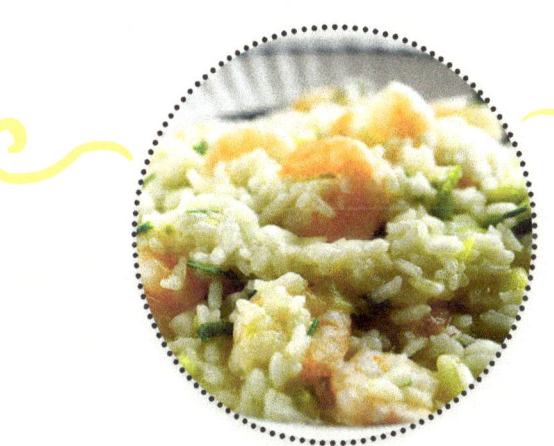

Chicken Curry

PREPARATION 10 MINUTES | COOKING 1 HOUR | SERVES 4

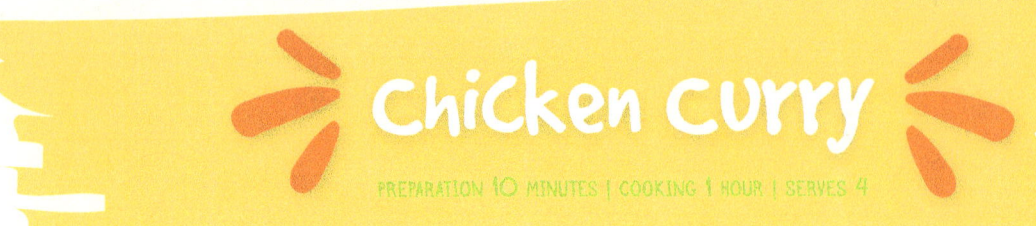

Ingredients:

Sunflower or vegetable oil (6 tablespoons)

3 cinnamon sticks

4 green cardamom pods

3 bay leaves

2 large onions, sliced

4 cloves garlic, crushed

Fresh ginger (4cm/1.5 inches), peeled and grated

Turmeric (1 teaspoon)

Chilli powder (half a teaspoon)

White vinegar (2 tablespoons)

Chicken breasts (600g), cut in chunks

Salt (1 teaspoon)

Sugar (half a teaspoon)

2 medium potatoes, cut into chunks

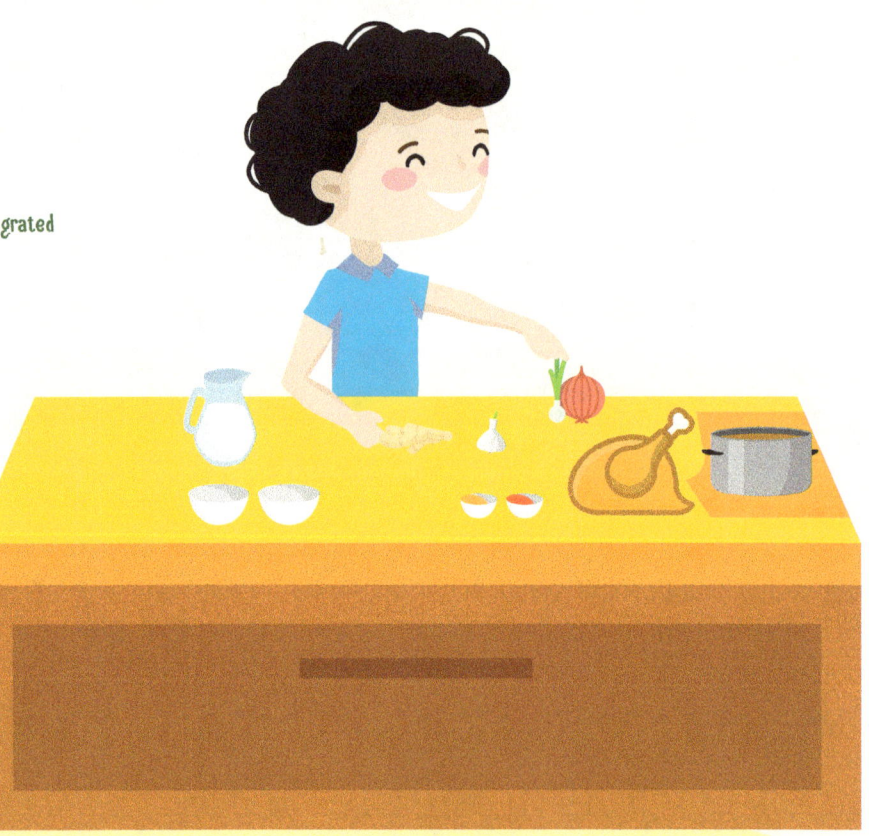

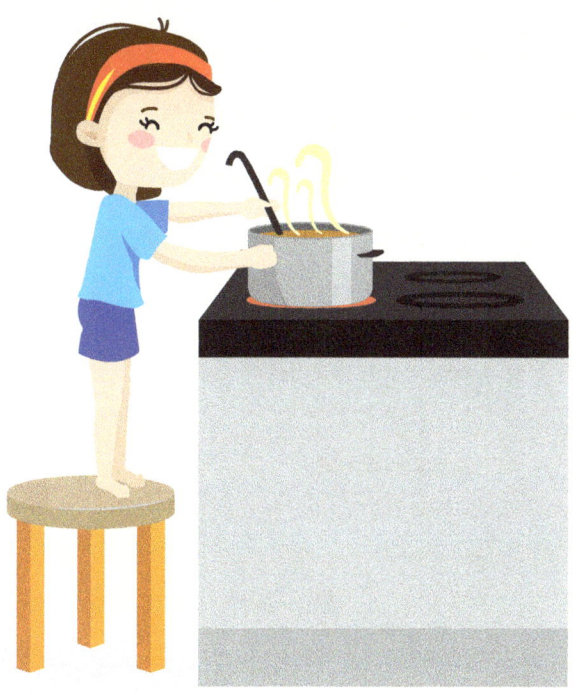

Method:

1. Heat the oil in a large pan. Add the cinnamon, cardamom and bay leaves and let them sizzle for a few seconds.
2. Add the onions to the pan and cook until soft and lightly browned. Then add the garlic and ginger and fry for 1 minute.
3. Add the turmeric, chilli and vinegar. Stir everything together.
4. Add the chicken and fry for 5 to 6 minutes until browned.
5. Once the chicken is browned, add the salt and sugar. Mix everything together.
6. Pour in 300ml of water and bring to the boil. Cover and cook on a lower heat for 15 minutes.
7. Add the potatoes and continue to cook for 20 to 25 minutes, until the chicken and potatoes are cooked through.
8. Serve with boiled rice, roti or naan bread.

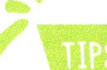

TIPS

If the curry starts to look dry, add a splash of water.

If you have a sore mouth, leave out the chilli powder.

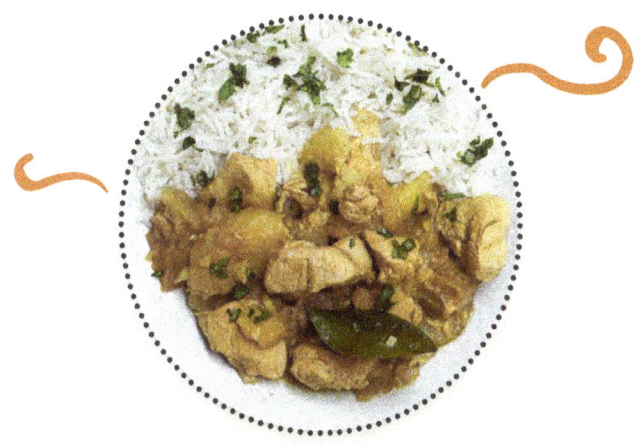

Quick Shepherd's Pie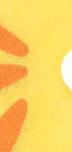

PREPARATION 10 MINUTES | COOKING 30 MINUTES | SERVES 4

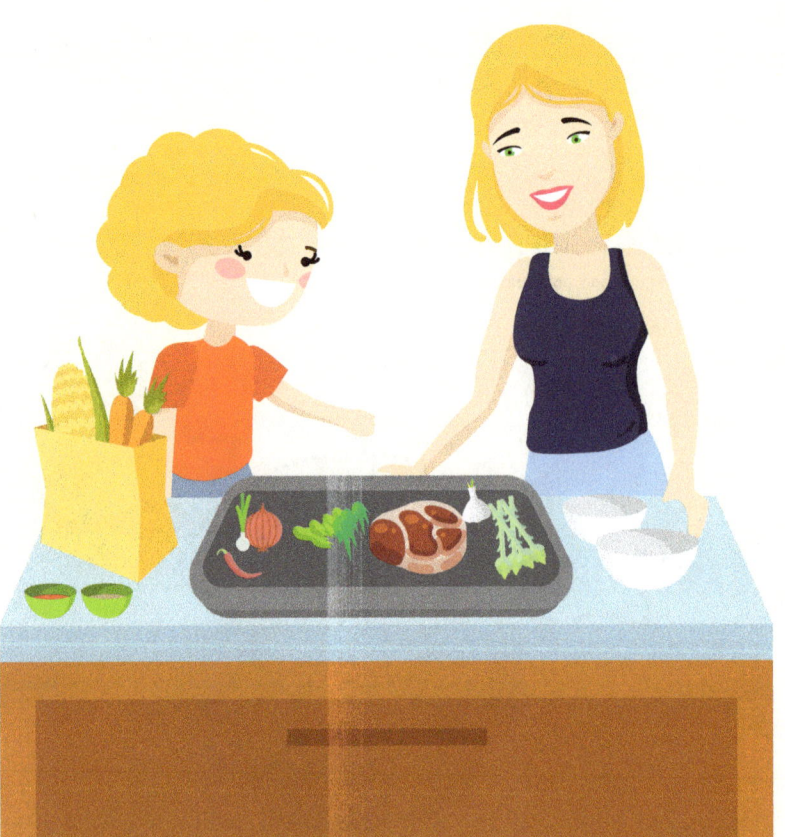

Ingredients:

Olive oil (2 tablespoons)

Minced lamb (500g)

1 medium onion, diced

2 medium carrots, peeled and diced

Dried rosemary (1 teaspoon)

Onion gravy granules (2 tablespoons)

Worcestershire sauce (2 tablespoons)

Frozen peas (100g)

2 frozen garlic baguettes

Method: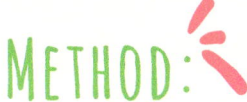

1. Preheat the oven to 200°C/180°C fan/gas mark 6.
2. Heat half the oil in a large pan. Fry the mince with the onion, carrots and rosemary for 5 minutes.
3. Add the gravy granules, Worcestershire sauce, peas and 85ml of boiling water.
4. Cover and simmer for 10 minutes, stirring occasionally.
5. Transfer the lamb mixture to an ovenproof serving dish. Slice the frozen garlic baguettes and arrange over the top of the mixture. Drizzle the bread with the rest of the oil and bake for 15 minutes until golden.

TIPS

If you have a dry or sore mouth or problems chewing, replace the garlic baguettes with instant mashed potato.

To reduce the fat content, use turkey mince or soya mince.

Speedy Moroccan Meatballs

PREPARATION 5 MINUTES | COOKING 15 MINUTES | SERVES 4

Ingredients:

Olive oil (1 tablespoon)

Ready-made beef or chicken meatballs (about 16)

1 large onion, sliced

Dried apricots (100g), halved

Ground cinnamon (half a teaspoon)

1 tin of chopped tomatoes with garlic (400g)

Toasted, flaked almonds (1 tablespoon)

Handful of fresh coriander, roughly chopped

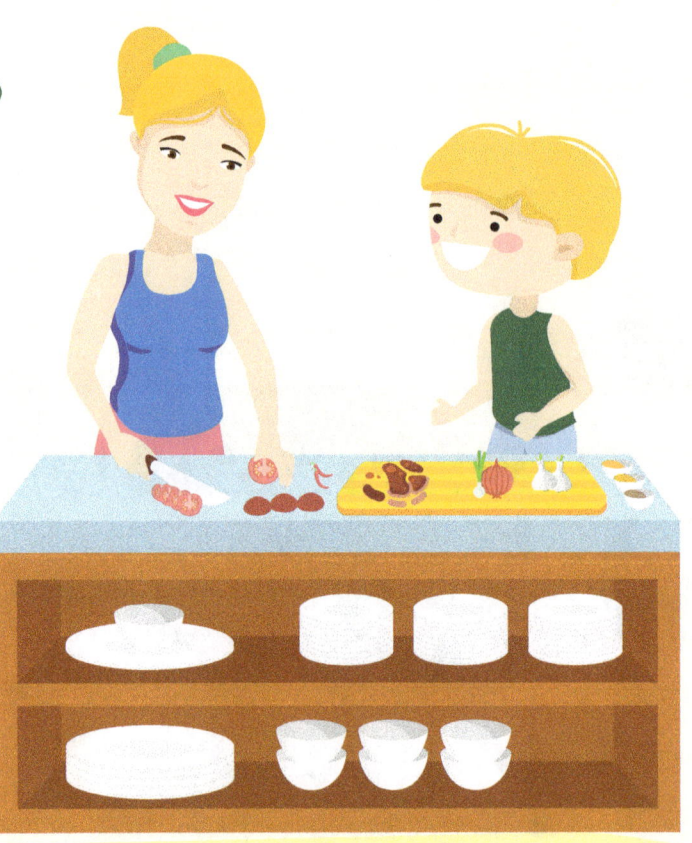

Page 96 MONSTER FIGHTING RECIPES

Method: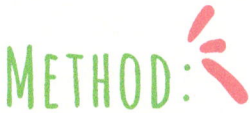

1. Heat the oil in a large, deep frying pan. Fry the meatballs for 10 minutes, turning occasionally until cooked through. Take them out of the pan and set aside.
2. Fry the onion for 5 minutes, until softened.
3. Add the apricots, cinnamon and tomatoes to the pan. Half fill the emptied tomato tin with water and pour into the pan. Stir and bring to the boil, then simmer for 10 minutes.
4. Return the meatballs to the pan and coat well with the tomato sauce.
5. Sprinkle with the almonds and coriander, then serve.

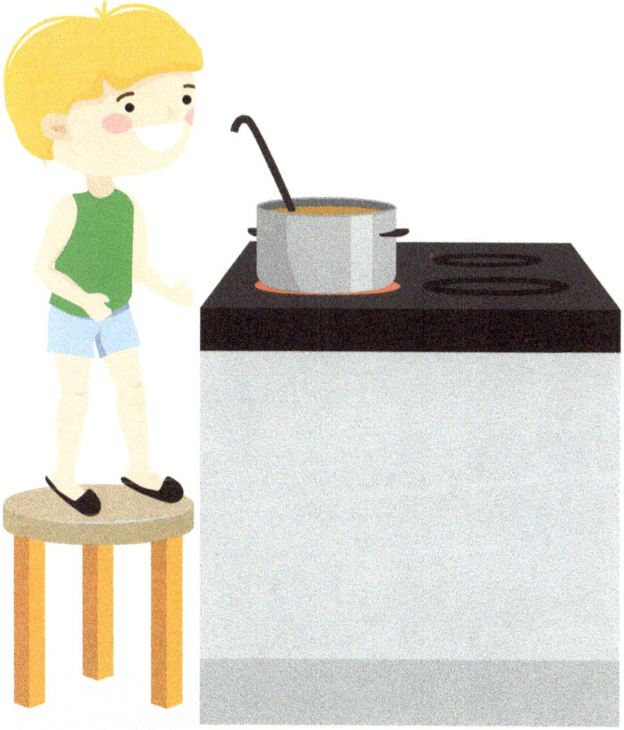

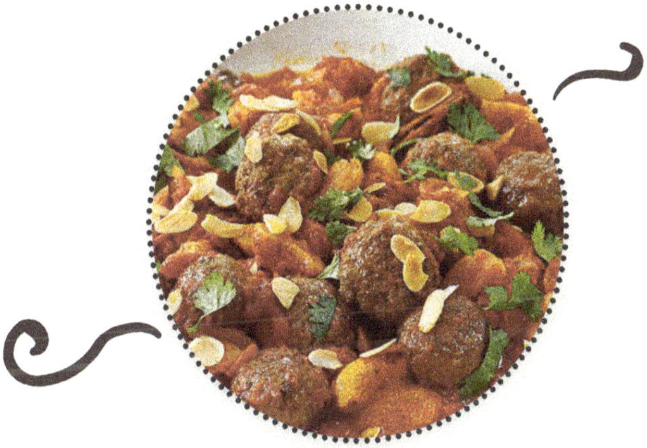

Butternut Squash, Raisin and Apricot Muffins

MAKES 12 MUFFINS

INGREDIENTS:

175g self-raising flour
50g brown sugar
1 tsp baking powder
1/2 tsp mixed spice
1 tsp ground ginger
100g butternut squash, peeled and grated
50g raisins
30g dried apricots, chopped
125 ml sunflower oil
75 ml maple syrup
2 large eggs

TRY THIS TASTY QUICK AND EASY MUFFIN RECIPE. YOU COULDN'T FIND A TASTIER WAY TO GET YOUR 5 A DAY AND THEY ARE FUN FOR KIDS TO MAKE THEMSELVES. THEY ARE ALSO DAIRY FREE.

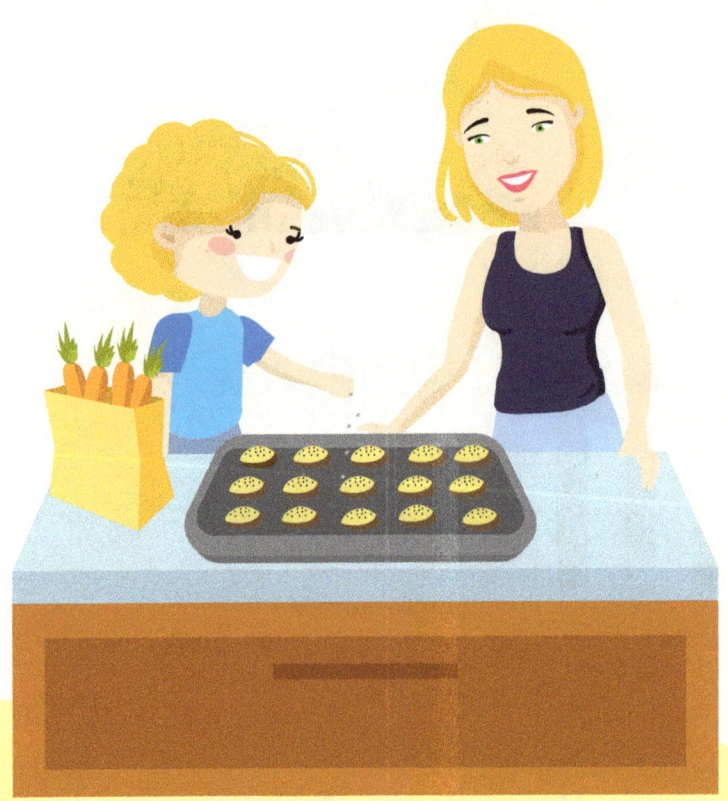

DECORATION:

Blueberries
Dried apricot

Method: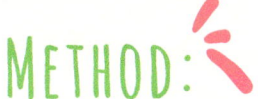

1. Preheat the oven to 180C Fan. Line a 12 hole muffin tin with muffin cases.
2. Mix the flour, sugar, baking powder, spices, squash, raising and apricots together in a bowl.
3. Mix the oil, maple syrup and egg together in a jug.
4. Mix the wet ingredients into the dry ingredients and beat together. Spoon into the cases. Bake for 20 to 25 minutes until golden and well risen. Leave to cool on a wire rack.
5. To Decorate. Make the ears out of halved dried apricots. Make a nose out of one whole apricot and half a blueberry and add blueberry eyes.

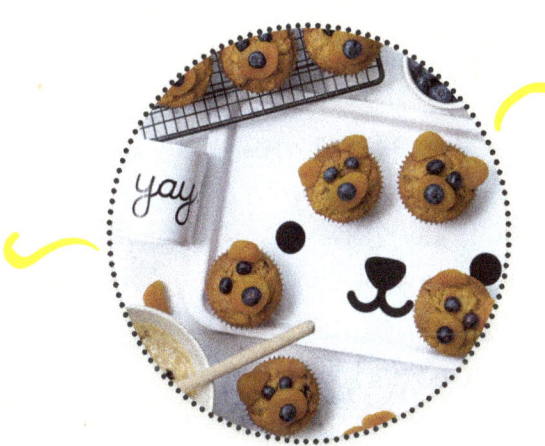

Spring vegetable casserole

PREPARATION 10 MINUTES | COOKING 30 MINUTES | SERVES 4

Ingredients:

Olive oil (2 tablespoons)

2 leeks, sliced

Carrots (100g), peeled and sliced

1 small swede or 4 small turnips, diced

2 garlic cloves, finely chopped

Vegetable stock (700ml/1.2 pints)

Salt and black pepper

1 tin of borlotti beans (400g), drained

Spring greens (150g), shredded

Pesto (2 tablespoons)

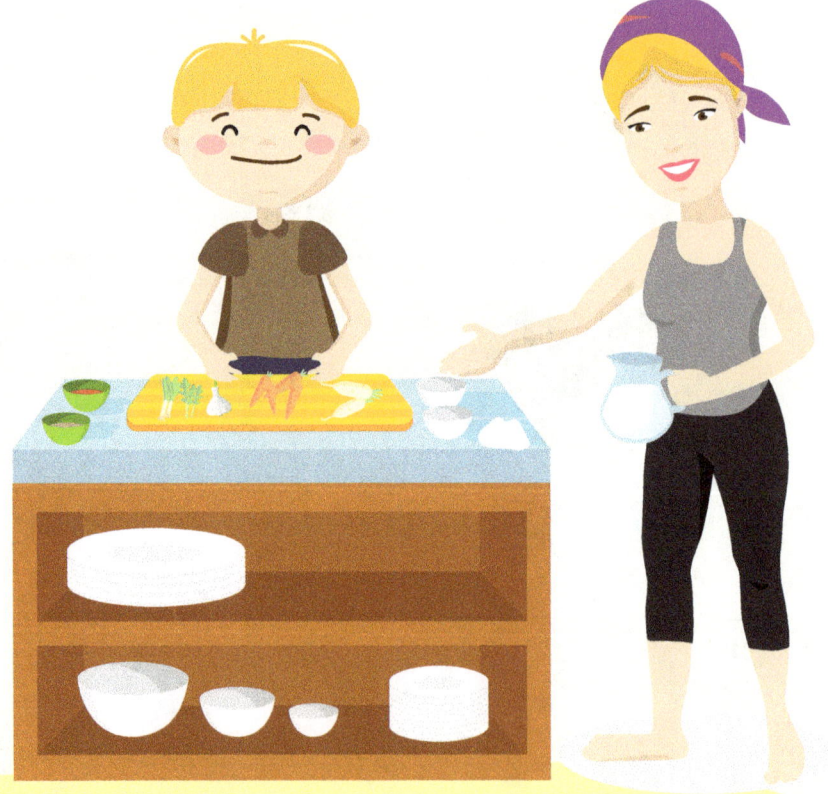

Page 100 MONSTER FIGHTING Recipes

Method:

1. Heat the oil in a large pan and add the leeks, carrots, swede (or turnips) and garlic. Fry over a low heat for 10 minutes, until the vegetables are soft.
2. Add the stock to the pan. Then add some salt and black pepper and bring to the boil. Cover and simmer for 10 to 15 minutes, until the vegetables are tender.
3. Add the beans and spring greens, then cover the pan and simmer for 5 minutes until piping hot and cooked through.
4. Stir in the pesto and serve.

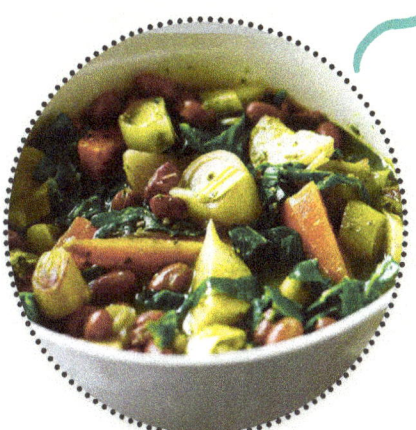

TIPS

For extra calories, serve with garlic bread or pasta.

Use a spray oil in a non-stick pan to reduce the fat content.

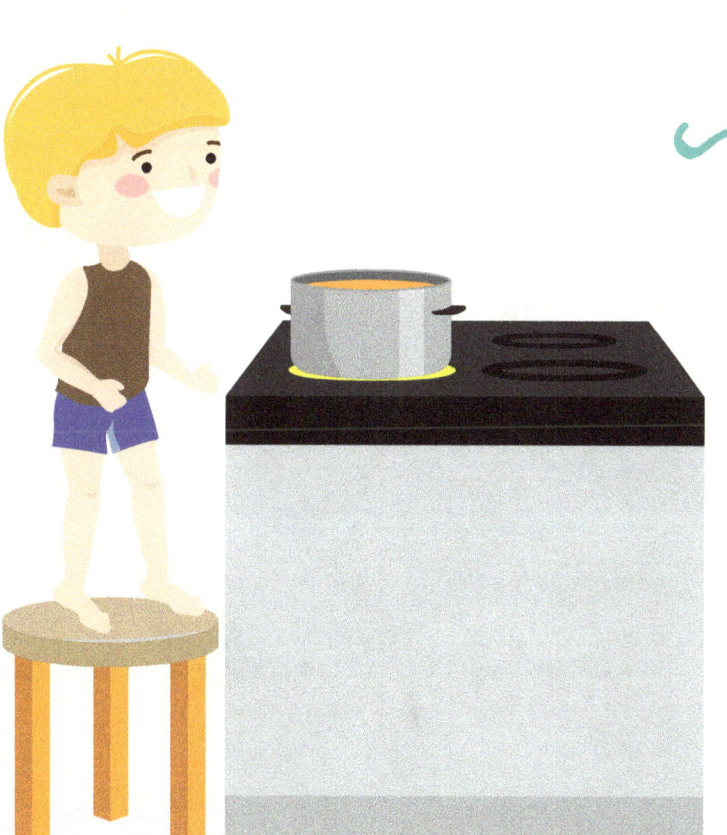

Mixed Bean Mexican Chilli

PREPARATION 10 MINUTES | COOKING 30 MINUTES | SERVES 4

Ingredients: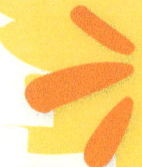

Olive oil (2 tablespoons)

2 cloves of garlic, crushed

1 red onion, chopped

1 red pepper, chopped

1 yellow pepper, chopped

Cajun seasoning (1 teaspoon)

1 tin of kidney beans (400g), rinsed and drained

1 tin of cannellini beans (400g), rinsed and drained

1 tin of chopped tomatoes (400g)

Vegetable stock (150ml)

1 tablespoon of dark chocolate, chopped

Handful of chopped coriander

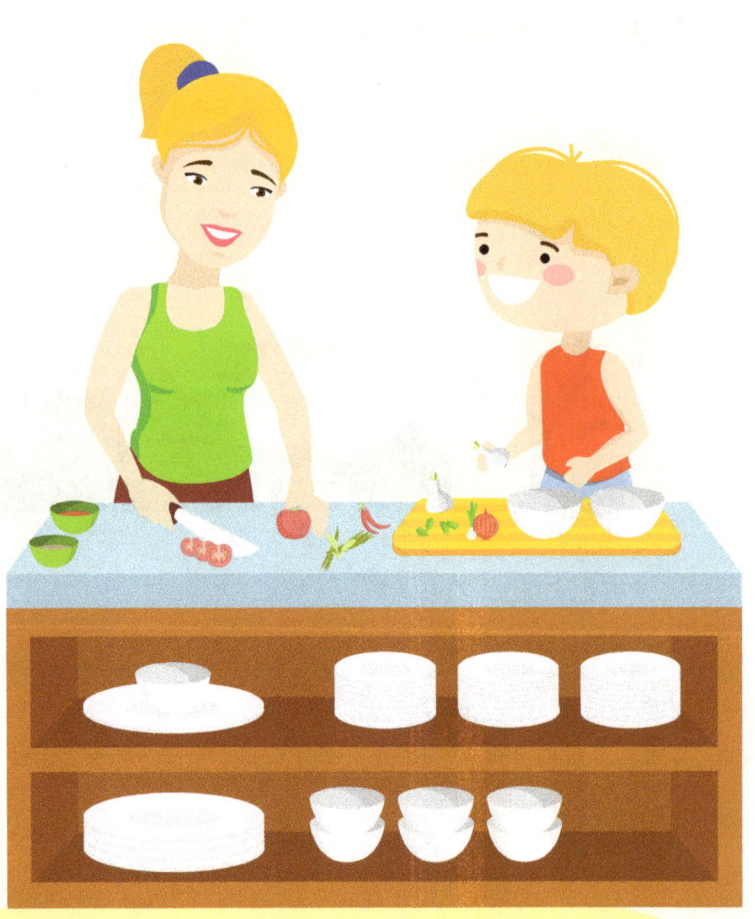

Method:

1. Heat the olive oil in a pan and fry the garlic, onion and peppers for 5 minutes.
2. Add the Cajun seasoning, beans, tomatoes and stock. Cover and simmer for 15 to 20 minutes.
3. Remove the pan from the heat and stir in the chocolate until melted.
4. Garnish with coriander and serve with rice, tortilla chips or potato wedges.

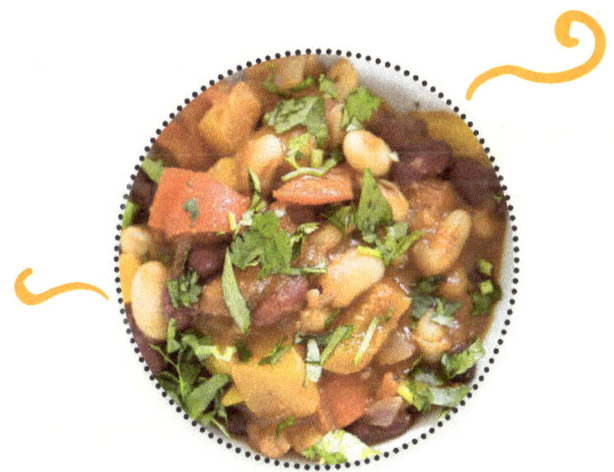

Fish Pie

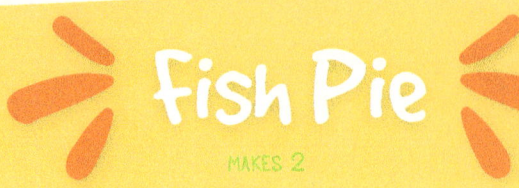

MAKES 2

THIS FISH PIE IS MADE WITH A TWIST WITH ITS FINISHING TOUCH OF SWEET POTATO, CARROT, PUMPKIN AND BUTTERNUT SQUASH TOPPING, ALL OF WHICH WILL BOOST IMMUNITY AND NOURISH THE SKIN. PACKED WITH ITS OMEGA FATTY ACIDS, VITAMINS AND MINERALS, THIS TASTY WARMING RECIPE, IS PERFECT FOR A GROUP OF FRIENDS OR A FAMILY MEAL.

You will need:

TOPPING:

- 2 x carrots
- 2 x sweet potatoes
- 1 x small butternut squash
- 1 x small pumpkin
- 50ml choice dairy free milk / homemade nut milk
- 1 x egg yolk (optional)
- Pinch of sea salt
- Fresh black pepper

THE PIE:

- 200g raw king prawns
- 1 x small fillet each of sea bass, cod, salmon, lemon sole, monkfish (your choice of fish)
- 1 x tablespoon olive oil or homemade butter
- 1 cup of petit pois
- 1 x shallot
- 2 x cloves garlic
- 3 tablespoons parsley
- Pinch of thyme
- Potassium broth / vegetable broth (homemade)

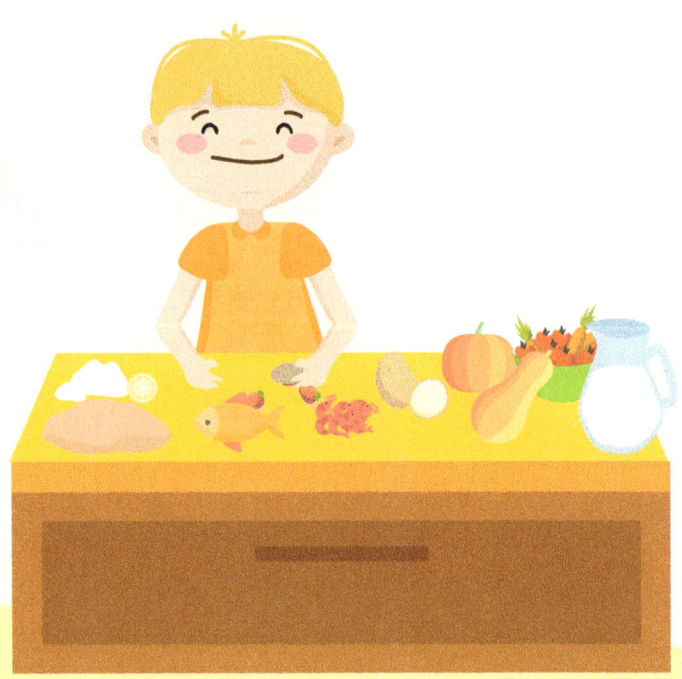

PAGE 104 MONSTER FIGHTING RECIPES

TO MAKE:

THE TOPPING:

1. Preheat the oven to 200c
2. Peel and chop the sweet potatoes, carrots, butternut squash and pumpkin
3. Boil until soft, drain the water
4. Mash and add the egg yolk, dairy free milk, sea salt and pepper
5. Mix until you reach your desired consistency – add a little more dairy free milk or olive oil if needed
6. Put to one side

THE TOPPING:

1. Whilst the potatoes are boiling, gently heat up some oil, and cook the fish and prawns in a pan with the lid on so that it cooks, softens and flakes
2. Add the peas, shallot, garlic and herbs and mix well, on low heat
3. Add the potassium broth or vegetable stock, add butter
4. Stir well and leave to simmer for 5-10 minutes

FINALLY:

1. Pour the fish pie mix into an oven dish
2. Add the topping
3. Place in the oven for 30-40 minutes or until the top starts to brown
4. Serve and Enjoy

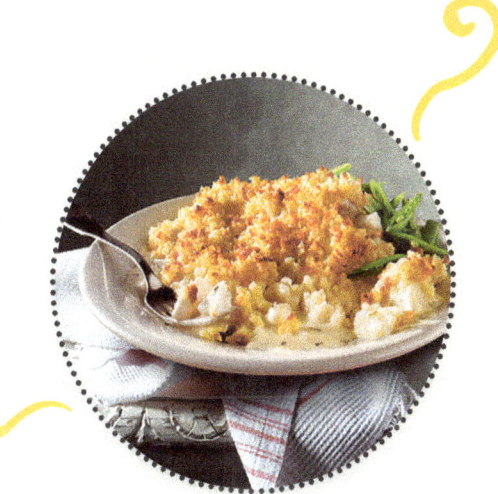

NUTRITIONAL VALUE:

A good source of vitamins A, B1, B2, B3, B6, B9, B12 vitamin that help to support the nervous system. Vitamins C, E, and K, iron, magnesium, potassium, copper, phosphorus, iodine, molybdenum, copper, choline, selenium, and rich in manganese which helps to boost bone strength the body's ability to process fats and carbohydrates. An abundance of antioxidants and anti-inflammatory properties which may help to boost your immune system, protect your eyesight, lower your risk of certain cancers and promote heart and skin health. The choice of sea salt contains 82 trace minerals, and can help boost adrenal/thyroid/immune system function. High in protein, dietary fibre and omega 3's, and containing ingredients such as Thyme which is great for stomach aches, sore throats and even bronchitis and Potassium broth which is a great source of hydration and immunity boost. Helps to alkalinize pH, help eliminate brain fog, improve memory, and ward off mood swings. Maintaining adequate potassium nutrition levels has also been linked to faster wound healing, diminished stress levels, lower blood pressure, and a reduction in age-related bone loss. Helps to flush system of toxins, poisons and unwanted salts and acids and give a concentrated amount of vitamins and minerals.

Stuffed Pepper Smiley Faces

Makes 4

You Will Need:

- 4 red/yellow or orange peppers
- 1/2 cup freshly cooked quinoa or sweet potato
- 8 baby tomatoes mashed or blended
- Small handful spinach
- 1 inch grated zucchini
- 6 asparagus spears
- 1 small shallot
- Thai seasoning – lemon grass, chili, garlic, coriander
- Cashew nut cheese (optional)

EVERYBODY LOVES A SMILEY FACE, AND THIS DISH IS FULL OF HAPPINESS, CREATIVITY AND VITAMIN C.

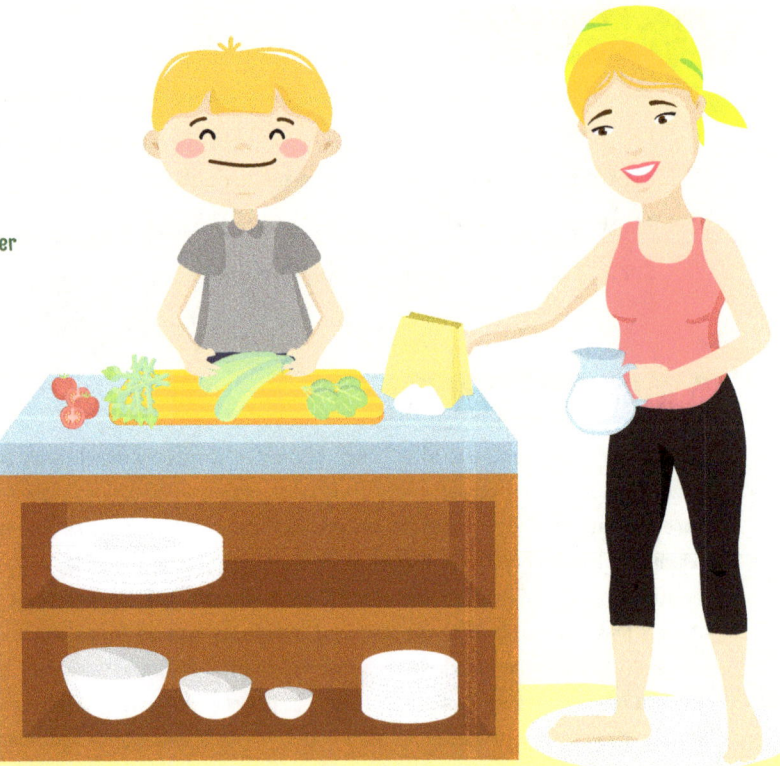

How To Make:

1. Preheat the oven to 200°C
2. Cook the quinoa or sweet potato
3. Wash and core out the peppers
4. Cut out some eyes, nose and a mouth
5. Place in a cooking dish
6. Blend the vegetables and herbs
7. Place the quinoa or sweet potato into a dish and mix in all of the blended vegetables and seasoning
8. Fill up the peppers
9. Top with cheese if desired
10. Place into the pre-heated oven for 20 minutes or until lightly browned on top
11. Remove and serve immediately

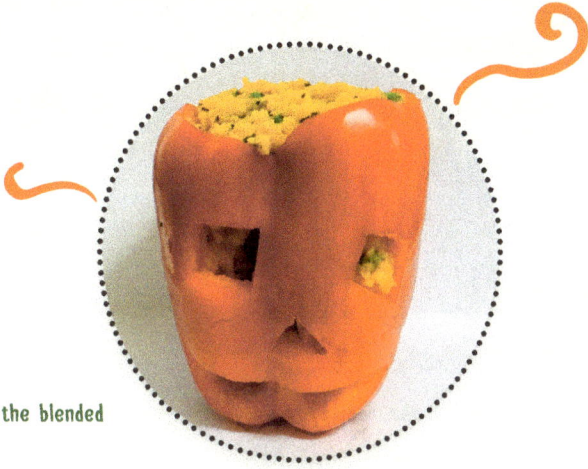

NUTRITIONAL VALUE:

High in Vitamin C, along with vitamins such as A, B6, B9, E, and K, minerals and macrominerals such as Potassium, magnesium, calcium, Iron, Copper, Manganese, phosphorus, chromium, choline and manganese. This recipe is high in protein and fibre, and even includes nine essential amino acids, with an abundance of antioxidants including lycopene, which has been linked to many health benefits, including reduced risk of heart disease and cancer. With ingredients that offer a good source of anti-inflammatory phyonutrients included in this recipe, and supporting the functioning of the nervous and immune systems, along with properties that have been known to help to relieve pain and swelling, reduce fever, improve levels of sugar and cholesterol in the blood, this recipe is delivered with a fun face appealing to children.

Mummy favourite fish Pie

8 PORTIONS

Ingredients:

600g peeled potatoes, diced

100g carrots, peeled and diced

A knob of butter

2 tbsp milk

25g grated Cheddar

40g butter

1 large or 2 small onions,

40g flour

400 ml milk

1 tsp Dijon mustard

1 1/2 tbsp fresh dill, chopped

2 tsp lemon juice

1 1/2 tsp rice wine vinegar or white wine vinegar

50g Cheddar, grated

25g parmesan cheese, grated

200g salmon, cubed

200g pollock, cubed

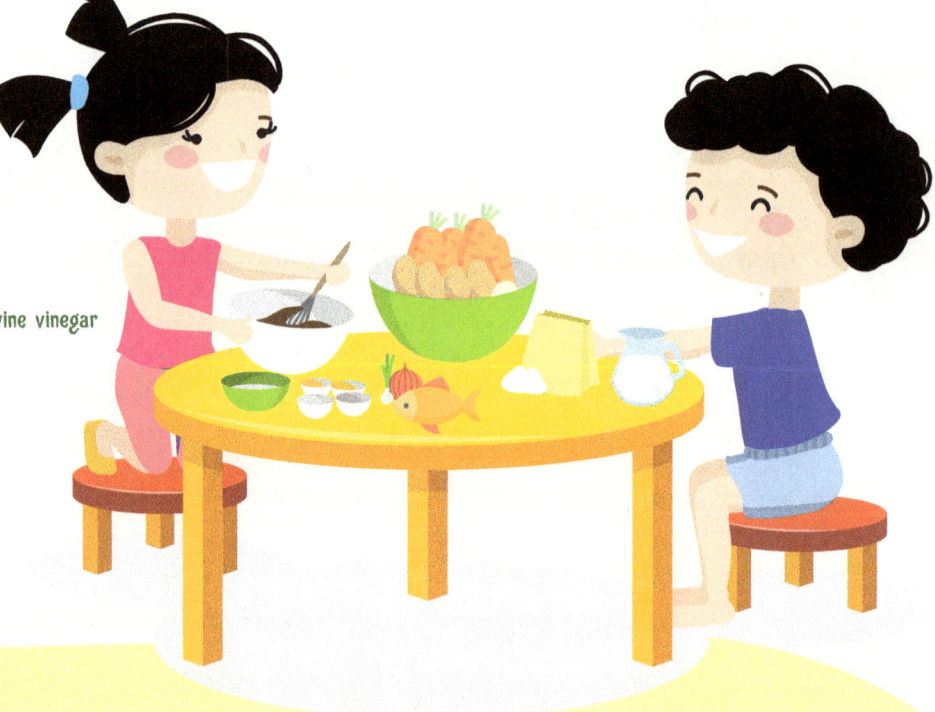

Page 108 MONSTER FIGHTING RECIPES

Method: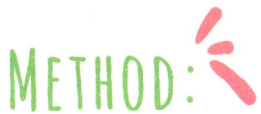

1. Preheat the oven to 180C Fan / 200 C / Gas 6.
2. Put the potatoes and carrots into a pan. Cover with cold water, then bring up to the boil. Boil for 15 to 20 minutes until soft. Drain, mash and mix with the butter and milk.
3. Melt the butter in a pan. Add the onion and saute for about 5 minutes until soft. Add the flour, then blend in the milk. Add the Dijon mustard, lemon juice, and vinegar. Stir until thickened. Add the cheeses, dill and fish. Season and spoon into an ovenproof dish. Top with the mashed potatoes and carrot and sprinkle with the remaining 25g Cheddar cheese for the topping.
4. Bake for 30 minutes until bubbling and lightly golden on top.

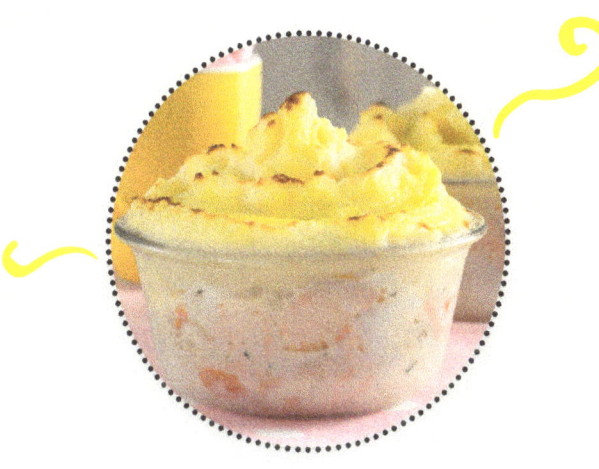

Hidden Vegetable Spaghetti Bolognese

MAKES 8 PORTIONS

Ingredients:

2 tbsp olive oil

1 small onion, finely chopped

1 small leek, thinly sliced

1/2 stick celery, diced

1/4 small red pepper, diced

1 small carrot, peeled and grated

1/2 eating apple, peeled and grated

1 clove garlic, crushed

1 x 400g tin chopped tomatoes

450g (1lb) minced beef

4 tbsp tomato purée

2 tbsp tomato ketchup

250ml (9fl oz) beef stock

1/4 tsp dried oregano

Salt and pepper

SUITABLE FOR FREEZING

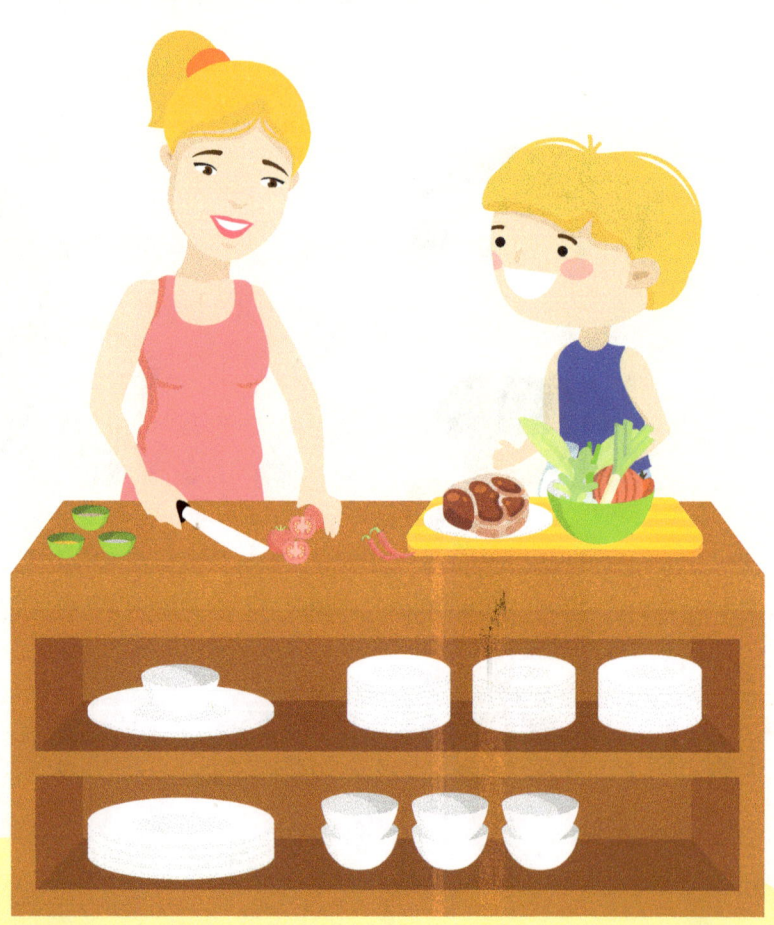

Method: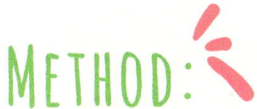

1. Heat the oil in a large frying pan and sauté the vegetables, apple and garlic for 10 minutes until soft. Transfer to a blender and add the tomatoes, then whiz until smooth.

2. Wipe out the pan with a piece of kitchen paper, then add the mince and fry over a medium-high heat, breaking the mince up with a wooden spoon, until browned (you may need to do this in two batches). If your child likes a finer texture you can transfer the browned mince to the food processor and whiz for a few seconds.

3. Add the tomato and vegetable sauce to the mince and stir in the tomato purée, ketchup, stock, and oregano. Bring to a simmer and cook for 40-45 minutes until the sauce is thick. Season to taste with salt and pepper.

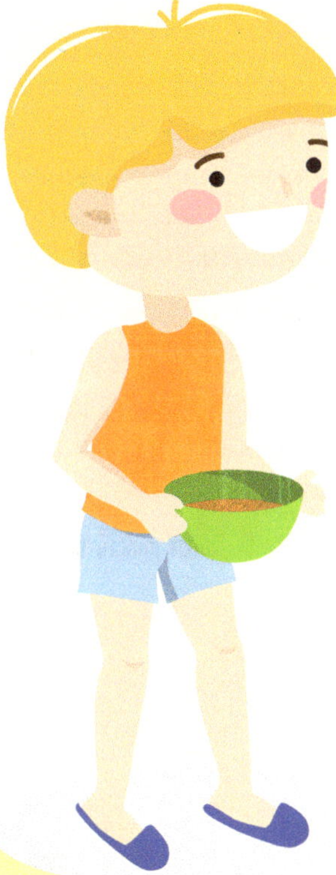

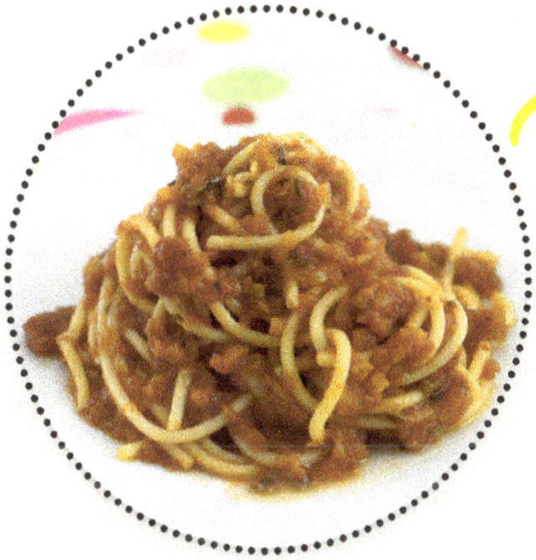

Tuna Pasta Bake

READY IN 45 MINUTES | COOKING TIME 40MINS | PREP TIME 5 MINS | SERVES 4

Ingredients:

500g Tomato and herb pasta sauce

300g Penne Pasta

3 x 120g tins of tuna in oil, drained and flaked

390g Chopped Italian tomatoes

325g tin sweet corn drained (optional)

100g cheddar cheese grated

2 pkts Salt and Vinegar crisps (smiths square being the best) Crumbled.

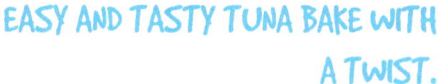

EASY AND TASTY TUNA BAKE WITH A TWIST.

Method:

1. Preheat the oven to 200c or gas mark 6.
2. Bring a large pan of water to boil and add the pasta, cook for 6 mins
3. In another pan pour Tin Tomatoes, tomato herb sauce and sweet corn (optional) and heat gently. Then add the Tuna flakes and stir as little as possible, keeping the flakes chunky.
4. Drain the Cooked pasta and add the Tuna and tomato sauce stir to cover pasta and then
5. Tip mixture into a 1 1/2 litre baking tray and sprinkle cheddar cheese and crushed Salt and Vinegar crisps.
6. Bake for 15 mins until golden brown and bubbling.

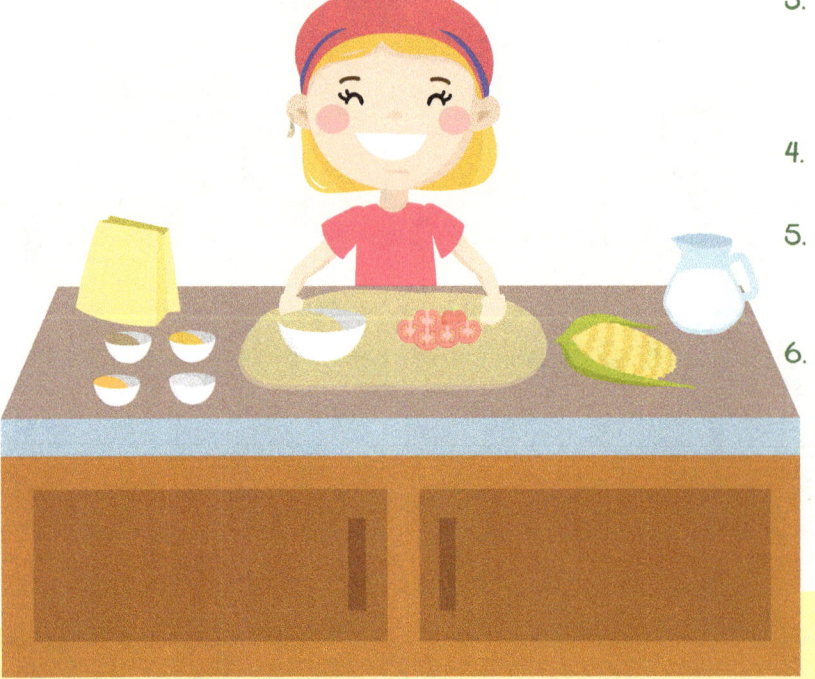

Page 112 Monster Fighting Recipes

ONE DISH CHICKEN AND RICE BAKE

READY IN 45 MINUTES | COOKING TIME 40 MINS | PREP TIME 5 MINS | SERVES 4

Ingredients:

1 can cream of chicken soup

340g: Chicken thighs

570 ml: Chicken stock

540g: mixed Frozen veg or fresh diced veg (dependent on timing)

Additional Water if needed

100g Cheddar cheese grated

EASY ONE DISH MEAL FOR THE FAMILY, I USE CAMPBELLS SOUP, BUT YOU CAN USE AN ORGANIC ONE OF YOUR CHOICE

Method:

1. Pre heat oven to 200c or gas 6;
2. Place chicken thighs in roasting dish, season and a splash of olive oil, bake for 20 mins until golden on top.
3. Once golden, take out of oven and place chicken to the side, in the same roasting dish, add the rice, cream of chicken soup, vegetables and one stock cube with water. Place chicken back on top of the rice mixture, and place back into the oven. Cooking times vary but generally speaking it should take 30 mins, the rice should have absorbed the water and be tender (add water if you find its dried out and rice is not cooked)
4. Add grated cheese and bake until golden brown
5. Serve

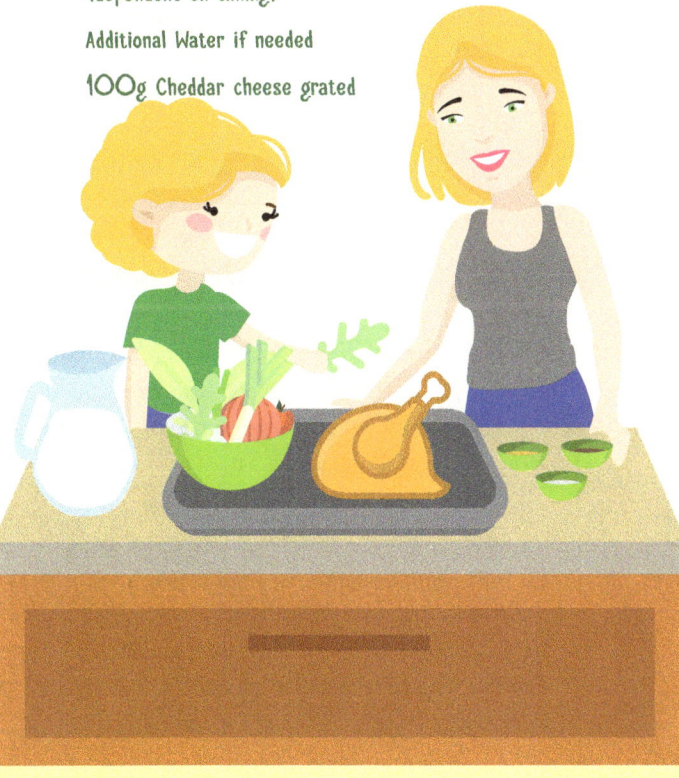

PAGE 113

Butternut squash lasagne

READY IN 45 MINUTES | COOKING TIME 40MINS | PREP TIME 5 MINS | SERVES 4

INGREDIENTS:

1 butternut squash peeled, deseeded and cut into slices

2 tbs olive oil

100g unsalted butter

100g plain flour

1 ltr milk

170g firm mozzarella cheese grated

50g parmesan cheese grated

Slat and ground black pepper

1 bag baby spinach (rinsed and drained) I personally use a lot more spinach at home:

Finely grated nutmeg

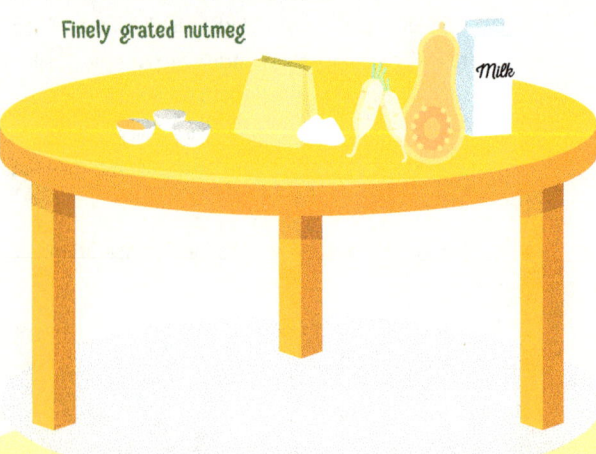

GREAT DISH THAT IS FULL OF NUTRITIONAL FACTORS

METHOD:

1. Pre heat oven to 200c / gas6

2. Gently rub a small amount of olive oil on the base of the lasagne dish, set aside.

3. Make bechamel sauce: Melt 70g of the butter in a large saucepan over a medium heat, sprinkle the flour over the butter and stir over the heat for about two minutes until flour is mixed in and cooked slightly. Slowly pour the milk over, whisking consistently. Bring to the boil gently while whisking keep whisking until thickened, season a little and reduce the heat to keep warm, stir occasionally to make sure its not sticking to the bottom.

4. Now place a layer of squash slices along the bottom of the dish, pour a layer of white sauce on top and sprinkle some spinach leaves, repeat, layer again with the squash slices and the white sauce and spinach and repeat.

5. Basically, you are substituting the lasagne for squash, the top layer should be white sauce and once in place, sprinkle grated the mozzarella and parmesan on top and cover with tin foil and bake for 40 mins, remove the foil and bake for a further 15 mins. (check the squash is soft to cut through as you would lasagne.)

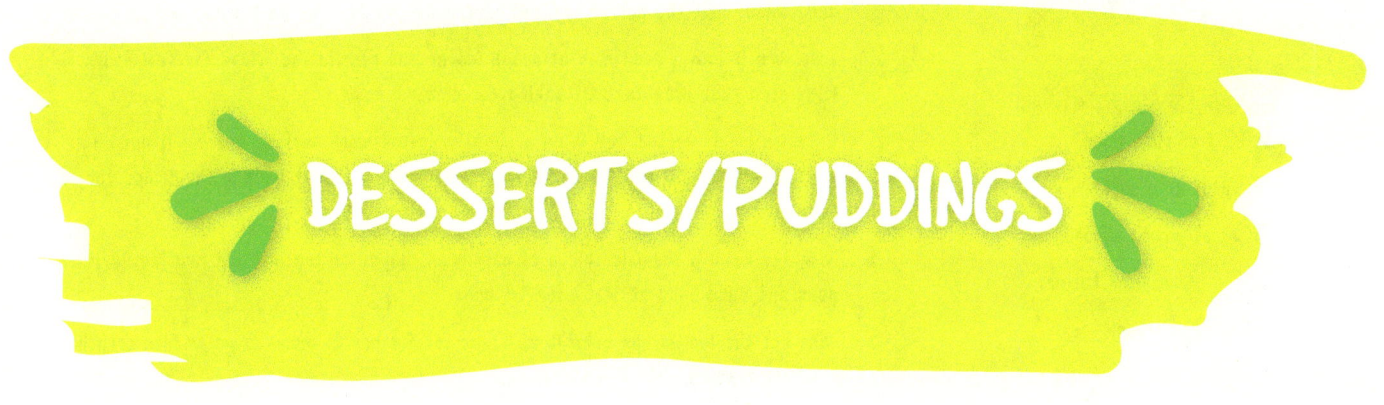

DESSERTS/PUDDINGS

Salted Sweet Potato Caramel and Chocolate Tart

STEP 1:

SWEET PASTRY-

- 240g of plain flour
- 90g of icing sugar
- 30g of ground almonds
- 120g of unsalted butter
- 50g eggs organic
- Pinch of salt

1. Mix all the dry ingredients in a bowl. Once throughly mixed, add soften butter and make crumb like texture, using a hand whisk, slowly add eggs. At this stage it would be not evenly mixed- knock it on a work surface and knead slowly. The heat from the hand would melt the butter and the pastry will be hard to work with, but its doable.

2. Just turn it into a even slab of dough, cover and rest in the fridge for few hours, first step post breakfast (if baking for dinner).

3. Once its nicely rested, roll it on a slightly dusted work surface and lay it out on a lined (parchment mould). pierce it with fork and knock it back in the fridge for 10mins

4. Now, lay down a crumbled piece of parchment paper on top and add raw lentils/chickpeas and Blind bake at 160 for 14 mins.

5. Take out the lentils and bake it at 175c for further 6 mins, to get a nice crunchy yet soft texture.

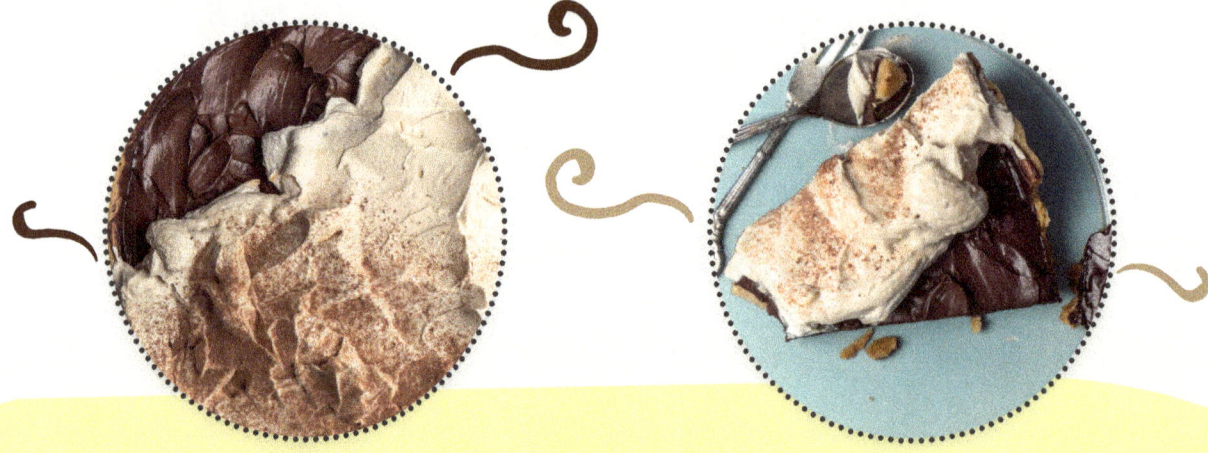

STEP 2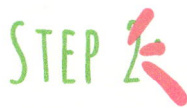

CARAMEL MIX-

Sweet Potatoes 150gms

sugar 50gms

butter 50gms

cream 125gms

Water 10gms

Sea salt- 5gms

1. Gently roast the orange sweet potatoes in preheated oven at about 175c for 25mins take the pulp out and set aside.
2. Starting from a cold pan, add sugar and water- gently increase the heat and achieve a nutty brown caramel. Don't be tempted to use a spoon while mixing the caramel- Keep turning the pan in circular motion to get all that sugar evenly melted. Water is a little cheat, makes it easier to work with at home. Now add the butter and whisk carefully, the butter all start to brown ever so lightly and the caramel would start to smell nutty.
3. At this stage, add cream and whisk on low to medium heat vigorously, in the beginning it would look split but carry on whisking and turns into a very shiny, beautiful tasting caramel. Finish with sweet potatoes and little sea salt.
4. Set aside at room temperature so it doesn't set, but reaches a workable temperature.

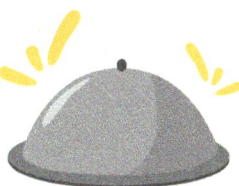

STEP 3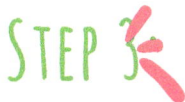

CHOCOLATE GANACHE FILLING-

Dark Chocolate 175gms

Double Cream 125gms

1. Bring the cream to just boiling point and pour over 150 gms chocolate. Mix using a spatula or a wooden spoon. You dot want to incorporate any air, so using a whisk isn't best. Once nicely mixed, add the remaining chocolate and bless your biceps with more mixing. Adding little chocolate towards the end, make it little more firm and gets a nicer texture.
2. Now, when the caramel and chocolate bot at room temperature- mix 1/3rd caramel with chocolate mix and stir nicely- a little marble affect is fine and works beautifully. Pour the whole mix in tart and using back of spoon create wave texture.

STEP 4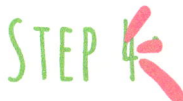

WHIPPED CREAM-

100gms double cream

Whip till get stiff peaks and mix in the remain caramel, spoon the cream over caramel chocolate and add loads of it.

STEP 5:

THE BEST ONE-

Let it set in the fridge and voila. xx

PAGE 117

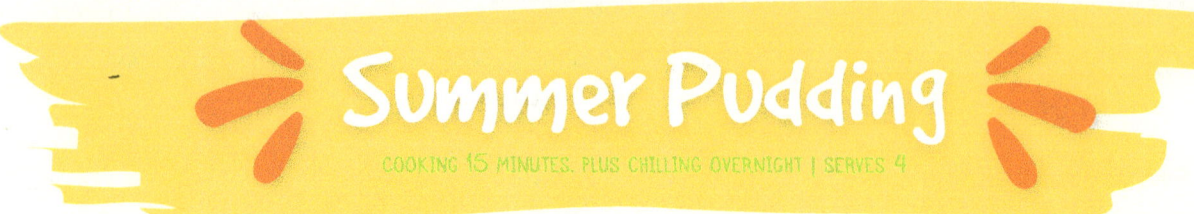

Summer Pudding

COOKING 15 MINUTES, PLUS CHILLING OVERNIGHT | SERVES 4

Ingredients:

Mixed fruits – raspberries, blackberries, redcurrants and blackcurrants (900g in total)

Caster sugar (115g)

Juice of a lemon

1 cinnamon stick

Bread (450g), one day old, sliced and crusts removed

Clotted cream (150ml)

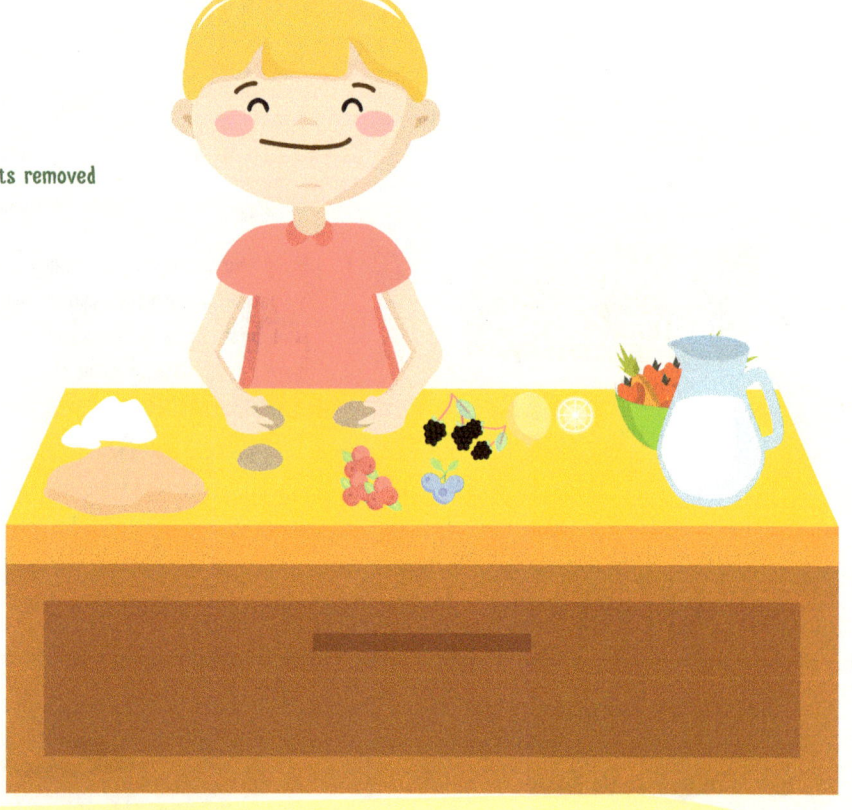

Page 118 MONSTER FIGHTING Recipes

Method: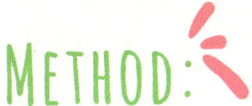

1. Wash the fruit and place in a pan.
2. Add the sugar, lemon juice and cinnamon. Bring to the boil and simmer gently for 5 minutes.
3. Use a colander and a bowl to separate the fruit from the juice. Put the fruit to one side.
4. Return the juice to the heat and simmer until it is reduced by half. Leave to cool.
5. Dip the bread in the juice, then use the slices to line the base and sides of a pudding basin or pie dish. Overlap the slices so there are no gaps.
6. Cover the base with a layer of fruit, then a layer of dipped bread. Repeat until the dish is full, ending with a layer of bread. You can keep leftover fruit or juice in the fridge for later.
7. Put a piece of greaseproof paper on top, and weigh it down lightly. You can use a plate that fits inside the rim of the bowl with cans or a kitchen weight on top.
8. Leave in the fridge overnight. To serve, remove the weight, paper and plate. Then, place a large plate upside down on top of the bowl and turn it quickly upside down, making sure the pudding has come out completely.
9. Serve with clotted cream and any leftover juice or extra fruit.

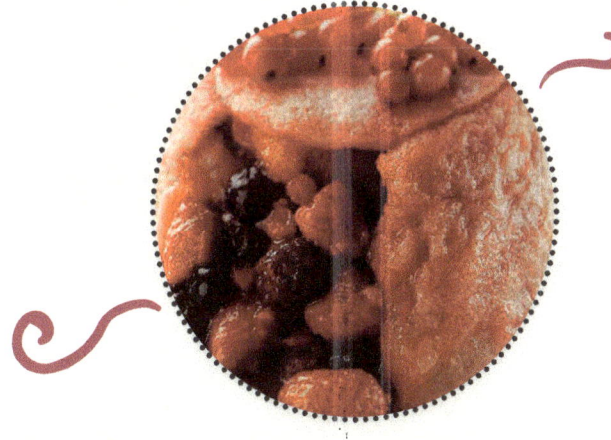

TIPS

To reduce the fat content, replace the clotted cream with low-fat natural yoghurt or fromage frais.

If you have sickness, leave out the clotted cream. If the fruit is out of season, buy frozen fruit.

PAGE 119

Greek Honey Cheesecake with Apricot Compote

PREPARATION 15 MINUTES | COOKING 35 MINUTES | SERVES 3

Ingredients:

8 digestive biscuits
Butter (56g)
Runny honey (2 tablespoons)
Curd cheese or ricotta cheese (225g)
Caster sugar (55g)
2 eggs, yolks and whites separated
Dried apricots (115g), chopped
Set honey (2 tablespoons)

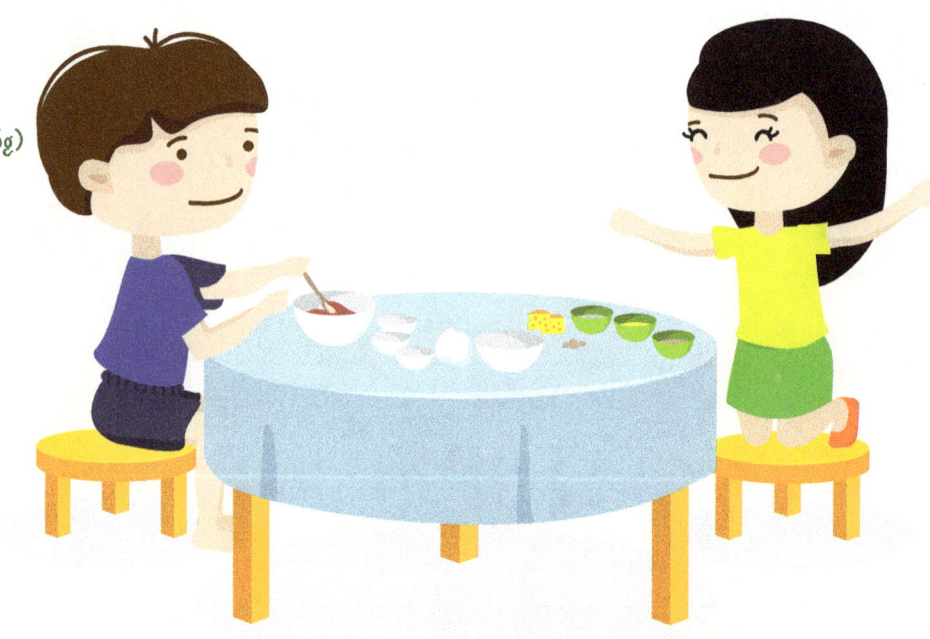

Method:

1. Preheat the oven to 180°C/160°C fan/gas mark 4.
2. Put the digestive biscuits in a clean plastic bag or freezer bag and crush into fine crumbs using a rolling pin.
3. Melt half the butter in a pan, then mix in the biscuit crumbs.
4. Use the mixture to cover the bottoms of individual ramekins or one round, ovenproof dish (about 20cm/8 inches wide and 5cm/2 inches deep).
5. Warm the runny honey in a small pan or in the microwave. Pour it into a bowl and stir in the cheese.
6. Add the sugar and egg yolks, and beat well.
7. In a separate bowl, whisk the egg whites until they form soft peaks. Then fold this into the mixture.
8. Pour the mixture over the top of the biscuit base. Bake in the oven for 25 to 30 minutes until the top of the mixture has set. Leave to cool.
9. Melt the rest of the butter in a pan. Add the apricots and set honey. Cook for a few minutes, then leave to cool for 10 minutes. Then spoon on top of the cheesecake. Cool before serving.

TIPS

Separate the eggs using two bowls. Crack each egg over one bowl, keeping the yolk in one half of the shell. Move the yolk from one half of the shell to the other, letting the egg white fall into the bowl. When there is no white left, drop the yolk into the other bowl.

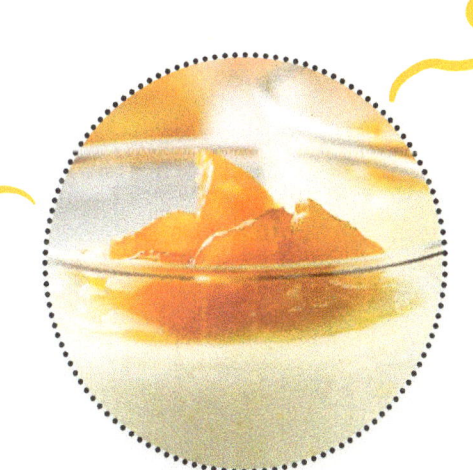

Brown Sugar Plums with Sour cream

PREPARATION 5 MINUTES | COOKING 25 MINUTES | SERVES 4

Ingredients:

8 plums, halved and stones removed
Light muscovado sugar (2 tablespoons)
Ground cinnamon (half a teaspoon)
Sour cream (300ml)
Demerara sugar (2 tablespoons)

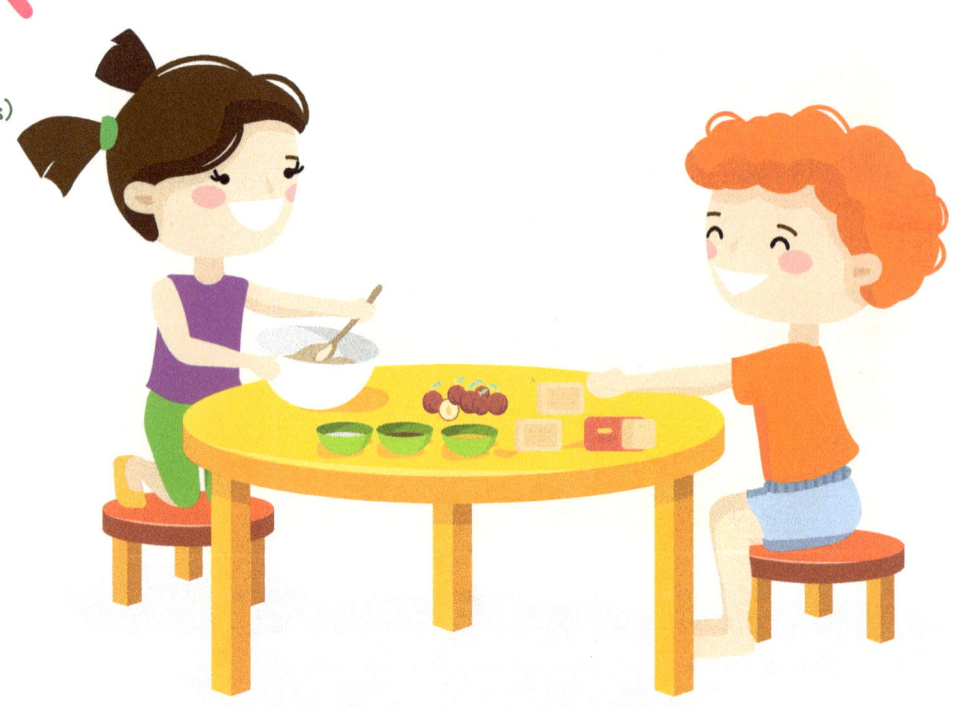

Page 122 Monster Fighting Recipes

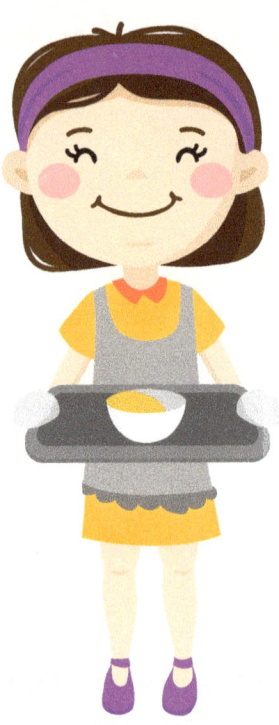

Method:

1. Preheat the oven to 220°C/200°C fan/gas mark 7.
2. Arrange the plums in the base of an ovenproof dish to make a tight-fitting, single layer.
3. Mix the muscovado sugar and cinnamon together, then sprinkle over the plums. Bake for 20 to 25 minutes until tender and golden.
4. Spoon the sour cream over the top and sprinkle with the demerara sugar.

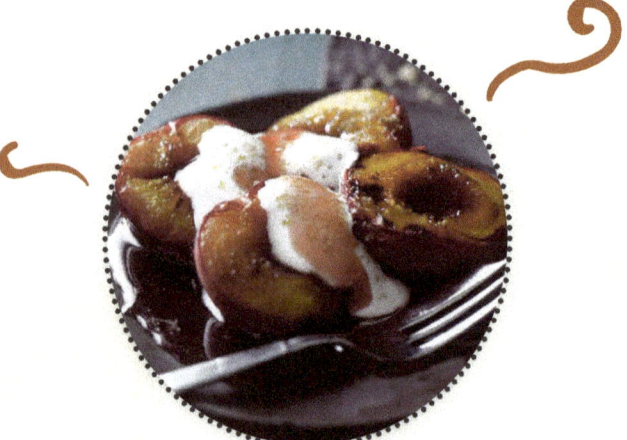

TIPS

For a crunchier sugar topping, put the dish under a hot grill until the sugar melts.

To reduce the fat content, replace the sour cream with low-fat natural yoghurt or fromage frais.

Microwave Banana Pudding

PREPARATION 10 MINUTES | COOKING 10 MINUTES | SERVES 4 TO 6

Ingredients:

Butter (100g)

2 ripe bananas

Light muscovado sugar (100g)

Self-raising flour (100g)

Ground cinnamon (2 teaspoons)

2 eggs

Milk (2 tablespoons)

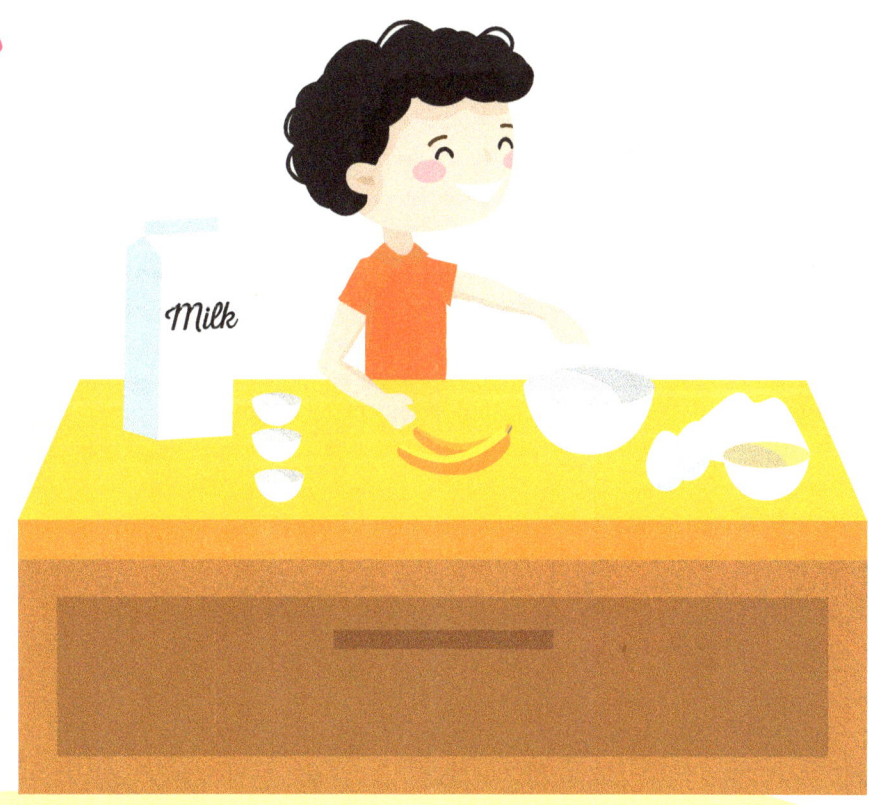

Page 124 MONSTER FIGHTING RECIPES

Method:

1. Put the butter in a 1 litre (2 pints) baking dish. Microwave it on high for 30 to 60 seconds until melted.
2. Mash 1 and a half bananas into the melted butter, then add the sugar, flour, cinnamon, eggs and milk. Mix together well.
3. Slice the remaining banana over the top, then put it back in the microwave and cook on high for 8 minutes until cooked through and risen. Serve warm.

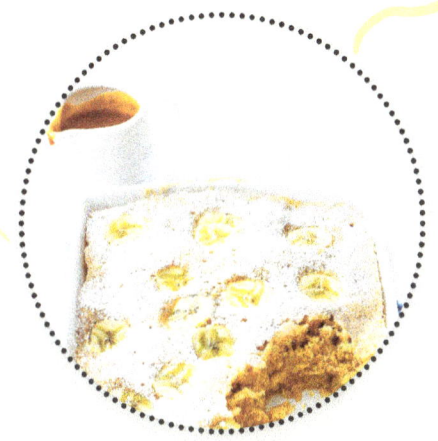

TIPS

It is best to use over-ripe bananas for this recipe. The browner and softer they are, the stronger the flavour will be when cooked.

For extra calories, try serving this with icing sugar, toffee sauce or a scoop of ice-cream.

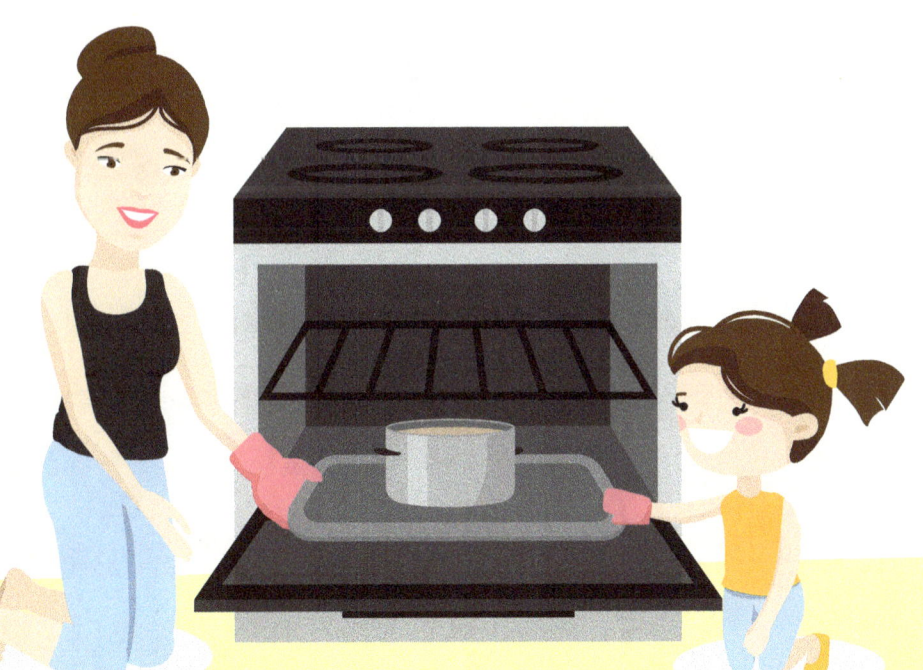

Coconut and Cardamom Rice Pudding

PREPARATION 5 MINUTES | COOKING 1 HOUR 30 MINUTES | SERVES 6

Ingredients:

Pudding rice (75g)

10 to 12 cardamom pods, very gently bruised with the end of a rolling pin

Grated zest of half a lemon or 1 small lime

Coconut milk (600ml)

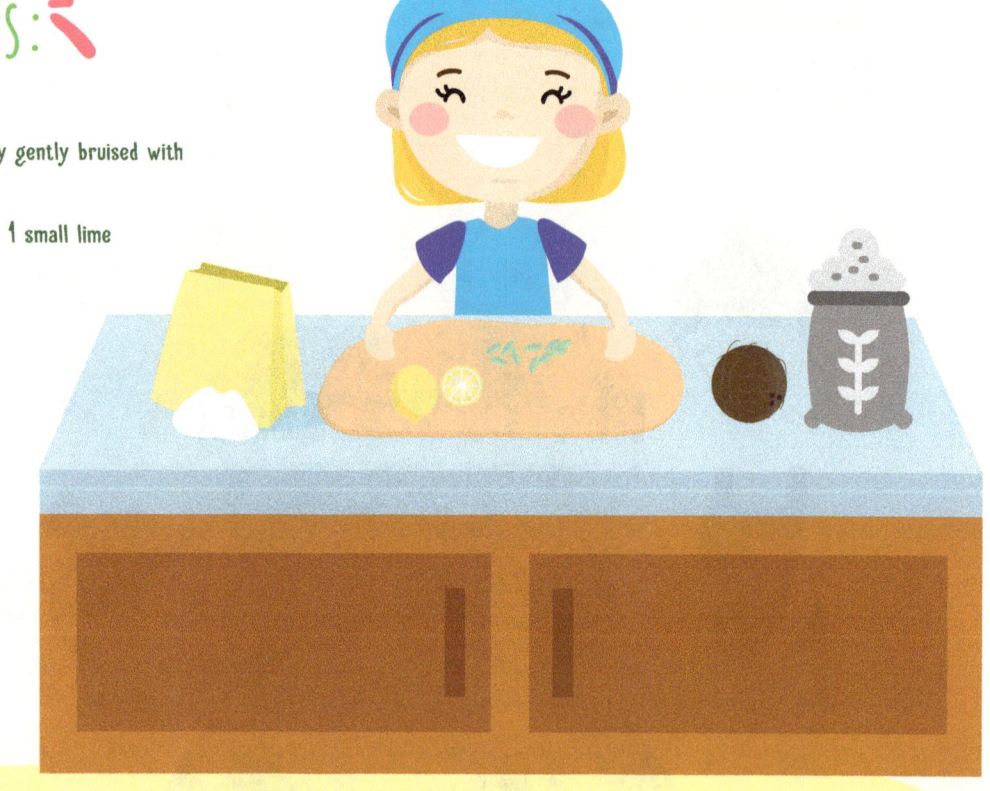

Method:

1. Preheat the oven to 150°C/130°C fan/gas mark 2.
2. Put all the ingredients in a shallow baking dish and mix gently.
3. Cover with foil and bake for 1 hour, stirring occasionally so that the cardamom is well buried to release as much flavour as possible.
4. After an hour, take the foil off the dish then cook for another 30 to 45 minutes, or until the rice is soft.
5. Serve warm or at room temperature, on its own or with fruit.

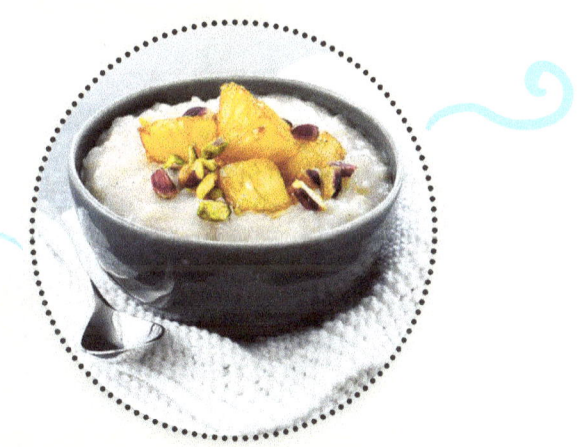

Amaretti Stuffed Peaches

PREPARATION 5 MINUTES | COOKING 20 MINUTES | SERVES 4

Ingredients: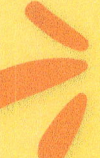

4 ripe peaches, halved and stones removed
8 amaretti biscuits, crushed
Mascarpone cheese (4 tablespoons)
Brandy or orange juice (2 tablespoons)

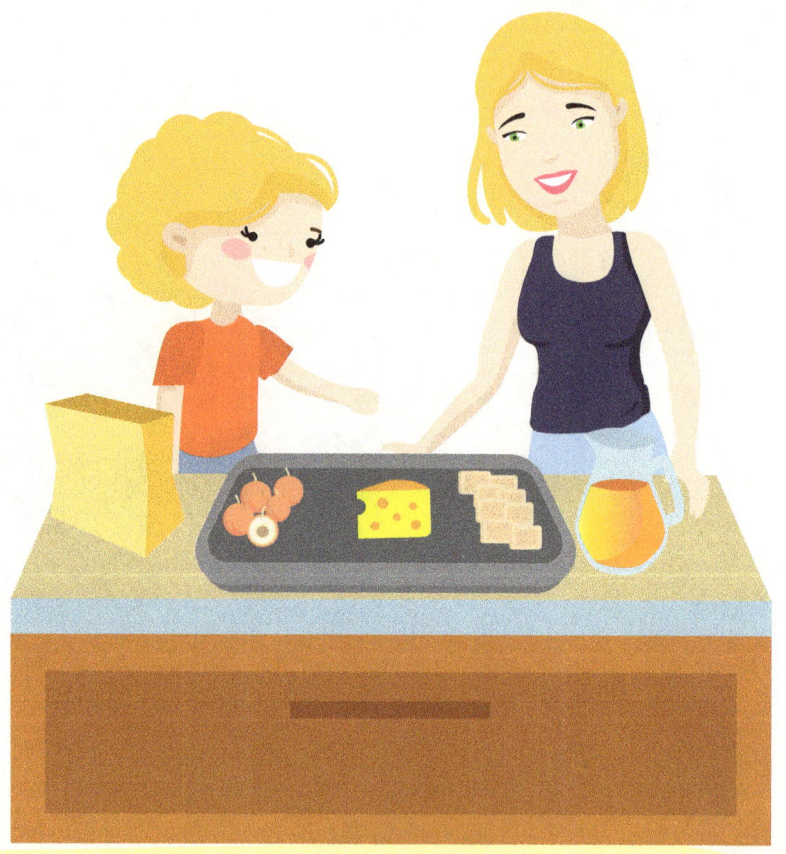

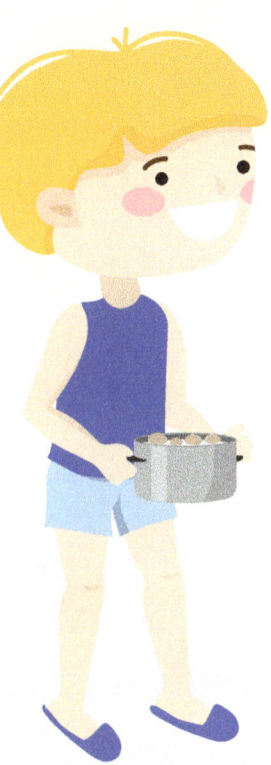

METHOD:

1. Preheat the oven to 200°C/180°C fan/gas mark 6.
2. Arrange the peaches in the base of a shallow ovenproof dish to make a tight-fitting, single layer.
3. Mix the biscuits with the mascarpone, then spoon it into the centres of the peaches. Sprinkle over the brandy or orange juice.
4. Bake for 15 to 20 minutes, until tender.
5. Serve warm or cold with vanilla ice-cream.

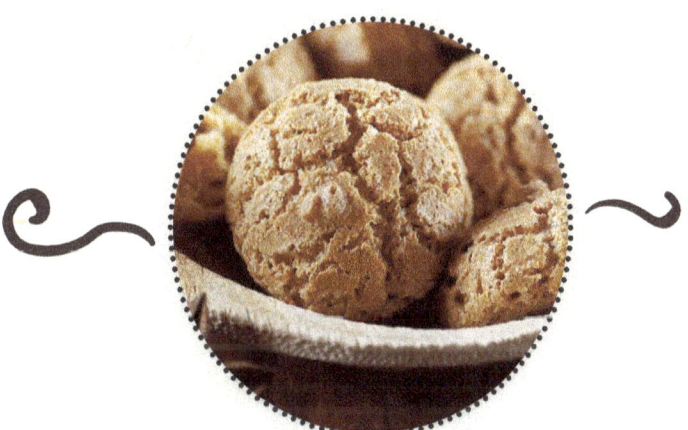

Beet Cupcakes
MAKES APPROX 25

You will need:

1 medium beetroot cooked and blended smooth

250ml hemp/coconut/almond milk

1 tsp apple cider vinegar

150g monkfruit sweetener or black seed raw honey

1 small avocado mashed

2 tsp vanilla pod seeds

250g of almond flour

100g unsweetened cocoa powder or 50g cacao powder

1 tsp Ceylon cinnamon

1 tsp nutmeg

1 tsp baking soda

1/2 tsp baking powder

1 pinch salt

GOOEY, NATURALLY SWEET, HEALTHY AND FULL OF GOODNESS I HEAR YOU SAY...?

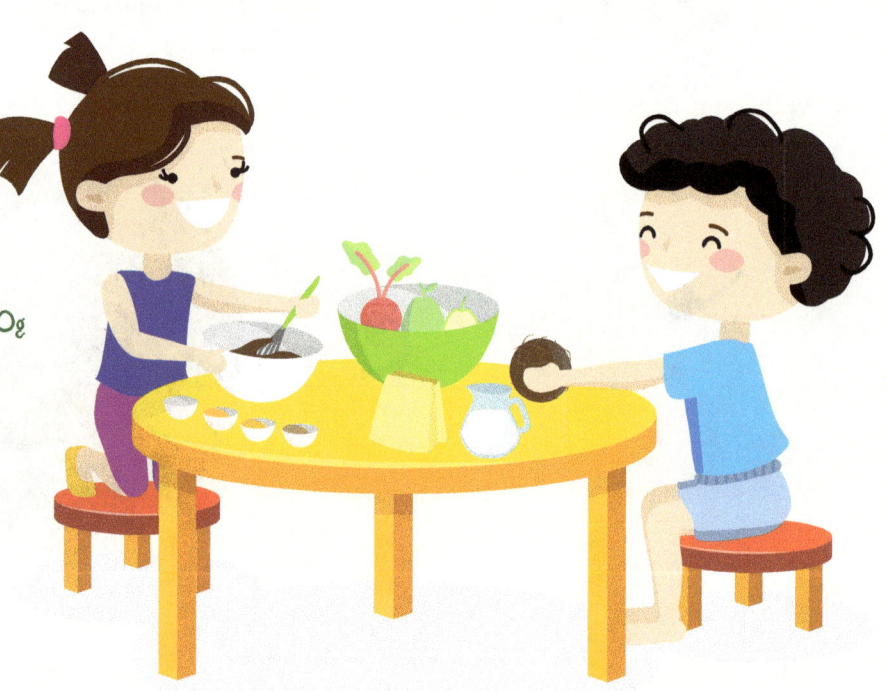

How to Make:

1. Preheat oven to 190 C
2. Line a cake tin or cake cases
3. Whisk together the milk and vinegar in a large bowl, then leave a few minutes to curdle.
4. Add the monkfruit, vanilla, and beetroot and mix until foamy
5. Add the remaining ingredients through a sieve, and mix until smooth – use a blender if possible.
6. Spoon into cases or pour into cake tin and bake for 25-30 minutes or until a knife test removes clean
7. Cool and either freeze for up to 1 month or keep in an airtight container

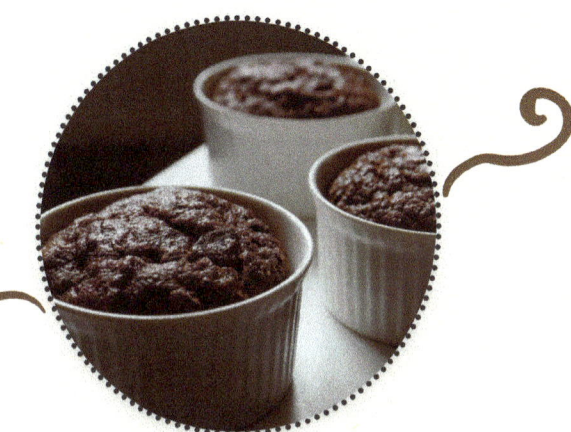

Nutritional Value:

Full of vitamins and minerals that help to protect your liver from toxins, and have been shown to have chemo-preventative abilities against some cancer cell lines, as well as thought to be free radical scavengers that help find and destroy unstable cells in the body. This recipe not only looks great, tastes great but is also full of absolute nourishing goodness. The nuts and seeds are high in healthy fats, protein, and fibre, some have Vitamin E, calcium, magnesium which is an energy mineral and vital electrolyte, and is associated with calming the body's nervous system. Antioxidants, amino acids and specific antioxidant properties from the apple cider vinegar have been shown to decrease blood glucose and up acetone level in urine. Rich in oleic acid, a monounsaturated omega-9 fatty acid, offer anti-inflammatory properties. This is a very well rounded recipe with energy boosting properties as wells as supporting the respiratory, digestive and immune system and containing ingredients that act as a natural antibacterial and antibiotic agent. For example Ceylon cinnamon offers Anti-oxidants, anti-inflammatory, anti-fungal, anti-diabetic, immune boosting, fibre, manganese and calcium in itself! And nutmeg is known for reducing joint and muscle pain, acting as a natural pain-relieving remedy containing a high quantity of myristicin, elemicin and eugenol. What a healthy cake recipe!.

Raw Honey Cookie Bites

You will need:

130g cashew nuts
20g tiger nuts
20g brazil nuts
20g hickory nuts
30g flaxseed or flaxseed flour
90g black seed raw honey
60ml coconut oil / almond oil / hemp seed oil or shea butter
115g monkfruit sweetener
1 tsp vanilla pod seeds
1/2 tsp cinnamon
1/2 tsp sea salt
Ach vegan dark chocolate
or cavalier dark chocolate
(cut into small pieces or grate)
*optional

EASY TO MAKE, TASTY TO EAT AND NO BAKING INVOLVED - SIMPLE

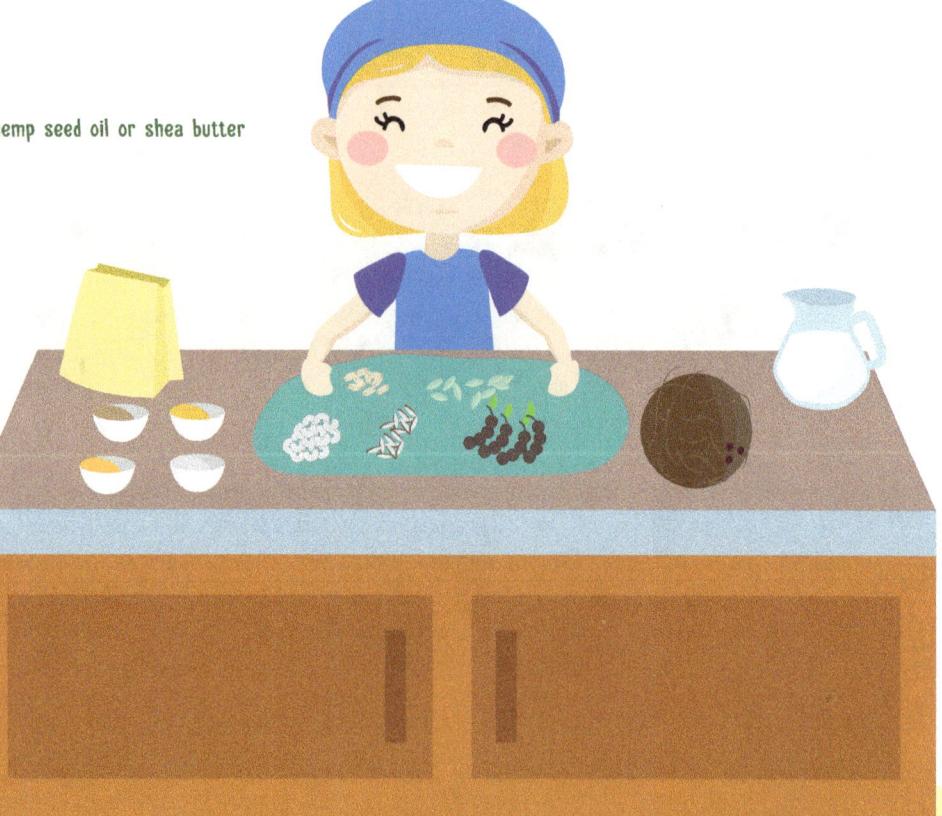

Page 132 Monster Fighting Recipes

How to Make:

1. Soak the nuts overnight in filtered water to increase bioavailability and remove lectins.
2. Blend the nuts down in a food processor until powdered/add flaxseed flour (or blend the flaxseed to powder too)
3. Blend down the sugar and add to the mix then add the vanilla pod seeds, cinnamon, sea salt, coconut or choice of oil, and honey.
4. Mix well until the mixture starts to become like a dough.
5. Add the chocolate shavings or pieces.
6. Put some into a glass container and use as a sweet nut spread, and roll the rest into balls.
7. Place the balls onto parchment paper and flatten to look like cookies.
8. Refrigerate for approximately 1-2 hours or until the dough sets.
9. Can be frozen and used later.
10. Will store in refrigerator for up to 5-7 days.

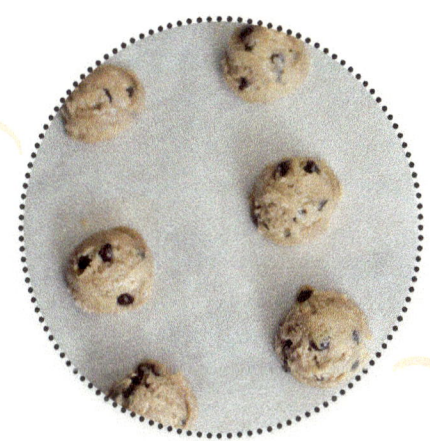

Nutritional Value:

High in healthy fats including Omega 3's and 6's, protein, and fibre, Vitamins A, E, F calcium, magnesium, iron, potassium, zinc, selenium, manganese, phosphorus, antioxidants, anti-inflammatory properties and more. Energy and Immunity Boosting, as well as possessing natural antibacterial, antifungal and antibiotic properties. Consuming higher cocoa content of 70% or higher, is associated with several health benefits, such that it may help to lower the risk of heart disease, reduce inflammation and insulin resistance, improve brain function, and provide more antioxidants.

Avocado Icecream

You will need:

350g Soaked cashews blended into a cream or full cream coconut milk

1 medium avocado pitted and peeled (scrape all of the dark green goodness from the inside)

70g or organic maple syrup or raw honey or monkfruit sweetener

1 tablespoon vanilla pod seeds

1/2 cup filtered water

(70g unsweetened cocoa powder or grated dark chocolate Ach or Cavalier) *optional

A DELICIOUS AND HEALTHY ICECREAM ALTERNATIVE THAT IS SUPER CREAMY AND DELICIOUS

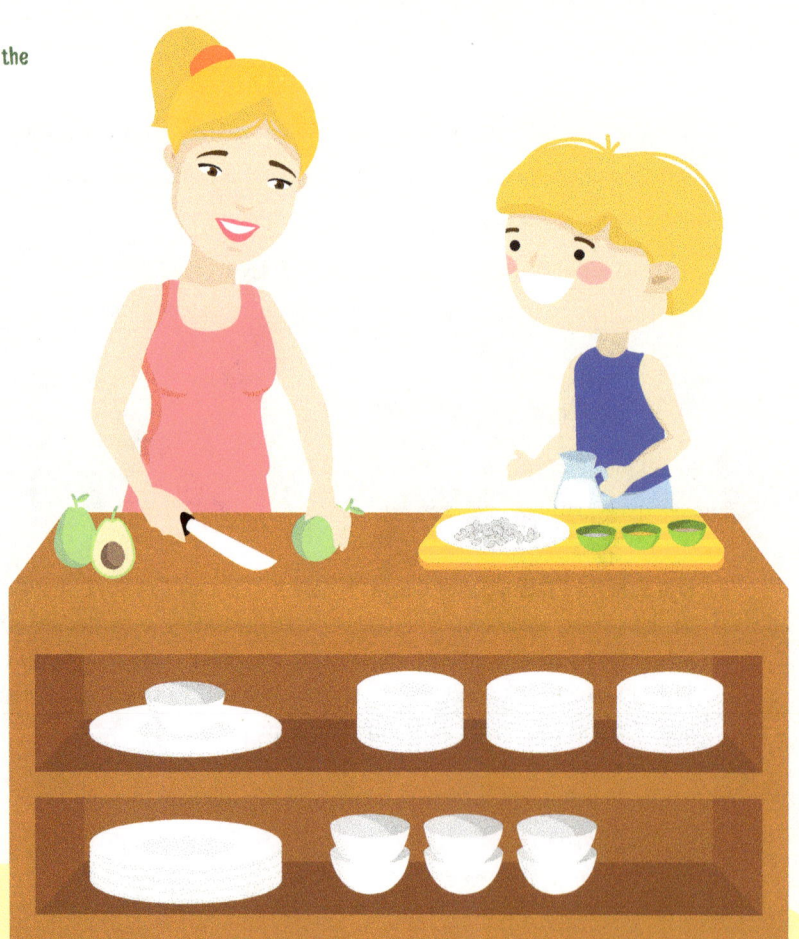

Page 134 Monster Fighting Recipes

How to Make:

1. Blend avocado and cashew/coconut cream
2. Add remaining ingredients and blend until smooth
3. Place in a glass container and allow to freeze
4. Mix every 20-30 minute for the 1st 4 hours as this will improve the finished texture by 100%

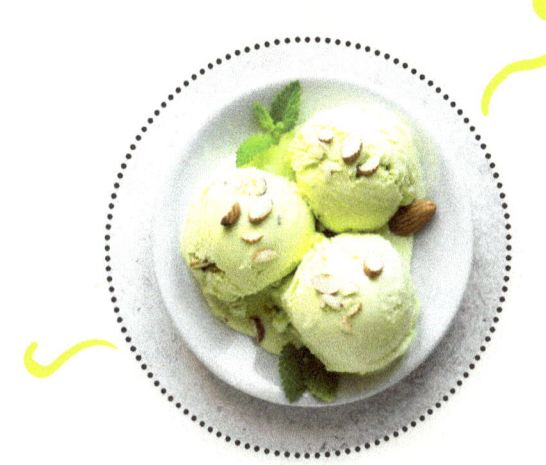

NUTRITIONAL VALUE:

High levels of iron, along with potassium, magnesium, zinc, copper, phosphorus, selenium and manganese. High in fibre, protein and healthy fats with anti-bacterial and anti-inflammatory properties. With the avocado this recipe will be and offering of *nearly 20 vitamins and minerals in every serving, including lutein, and a good source of B vitamins*. Consuming higher cocoa content of 70% or higher, is associated with several health benefits, such that it may help to lower the risk of heart disease, reduce inflammation and insulin resistance, improve brain function, and provide more antioxidants.

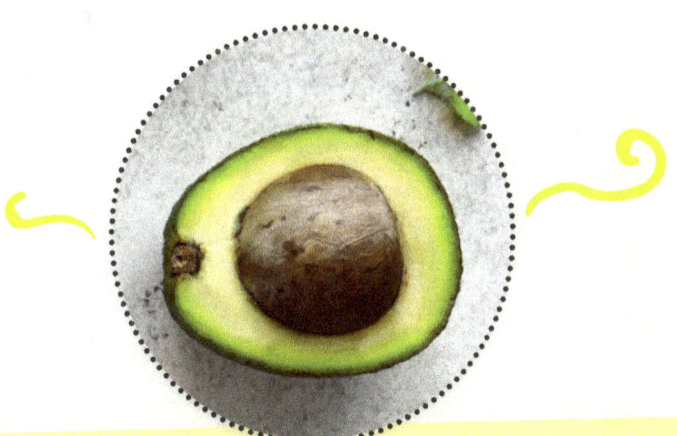

Raspberry Mousse

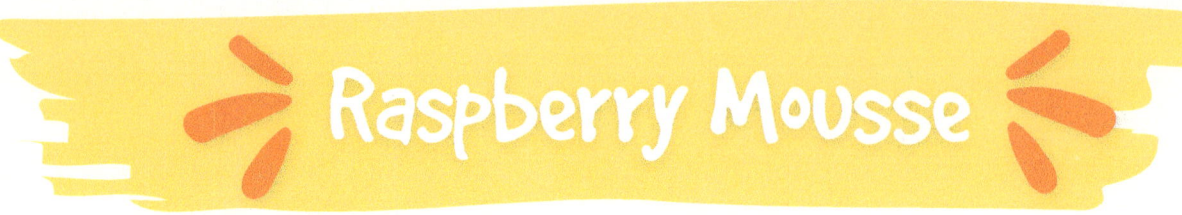

You will need:

250g fresh organic raspberries
160g cashew nuts
80ml marigold tea steeped for 10 minutes
50ml choice of dairy free milk
3 tbsp monkfruit sweetener
1/2 tsp agar agar vegetable glycerine

A HEALTHY, REFRESHING AND DELICIOUS DESSERT WITH A FLUFFY, SMOOTH TEXTURE THAT WILL IMPRESS AND SATISFY ALMOST ANY TASTEBUD.

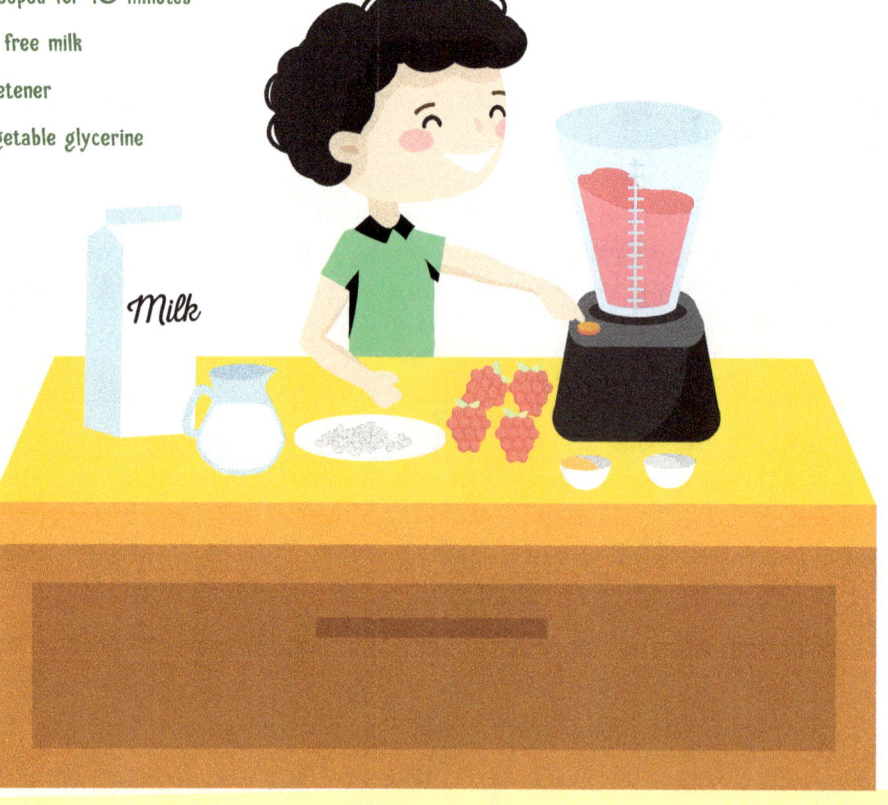

Page 136 Monster Fighting Recipes

How to Make:

1. Heat the agar agar gently in a pan until dissolved
2. Blend the raspberries, cashew nuts, water and sweetener in a processor until smooth
3. Add the agar agar and mix together for 20-30 seconds
4. (Optional – strain the raspberry seeds)
5. Divide mixture into 6-8 portions in glasses
6. Refrigerate until mousse thickens to desired consistency
7. Will store refrigerated for 2-3 days
8. Serve with fresh mint leaves / a sprinkle of ceylon cinnamon / a few fresh blueberries

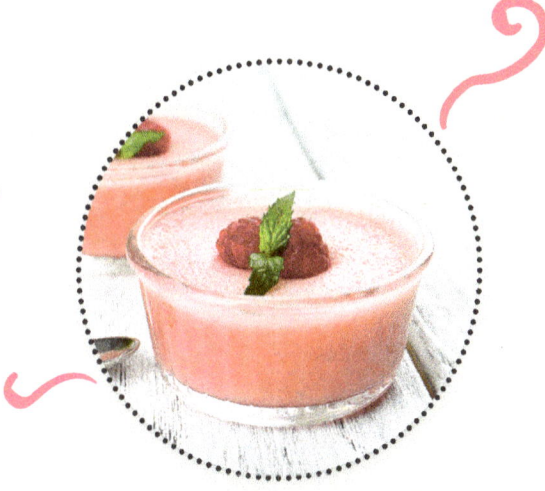

Nutritional Value:

Full of Strong antioxidants such as Vitamin C, quercetin and gallic acid that fight against cancer, heart and circulatory disease, and a known chemo-preventative, with anti-inflammatory and anti-oxidant properties. Calendula has also been used to treat leukemia, and cancers such as colon, breast and melanoma cancer cells. Lutein, an antioxidant extracted from marigolds, has been used successfully on breast cancer tumours. The results of studies show that lutein not only reduces the number of tumours in the breast, it also prevents new cancer cells from developing. Researchers have found that even in small dietary amounts, the lutein from marigolds have a positive effect. High levels of iron, magnesium, zinc, copper, phosphorus, and manganese

Lemon Mint and Ginger Lollies

You will need:

150ml freshly squeezed lemon juice

2 tbsp monkfruit sweetener or raw honey

2 tsp finely blended mint

1 inch fresh blended to juice

Ice lolly holders

2 tsp agar agar powder

LITTLE POWERHOUSES OF VITAMIN C AND ANTI-INFLAMMATORY PROPERTIES THAT ARE SURPRISINGLY EASY TO MAKE

How To Make:

1. Blend the mint, ginger and lemon juice.
2. Heat the liquid ingredient in a saucepan and add the monkfruit sweetener
3. Add agar agar powder and mix well
4. Taste – if needed add more monkfruit sweetener or raw honey
5. Pour into lolly moulds and add wooden sticks, or even make some creative ice trays as ice sweeties

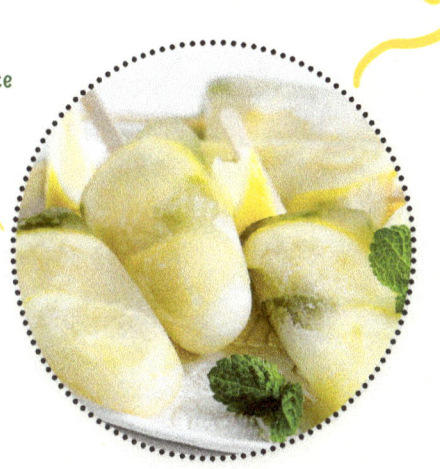

NUTRITIONAL VALUE:

High in Vitamin C, good amounts of B3, B6, B9, and small amounts of Vitamin A, potassium, magnesium, calcium, zinc, phosphorus, iron. This recipe can help to soothe digestion with ingredients shown to relieve pain and discomfort from gas and bloating. Peppermint tea is a common home remedy for flatulence. With ginger as an ingredient used in this recipe is can help fight infection, illness, inflammation, free radicals, cancer-causing molecules and is a great anti-inflammatory.

Page 140 MONSTER FIGHTING Recipes

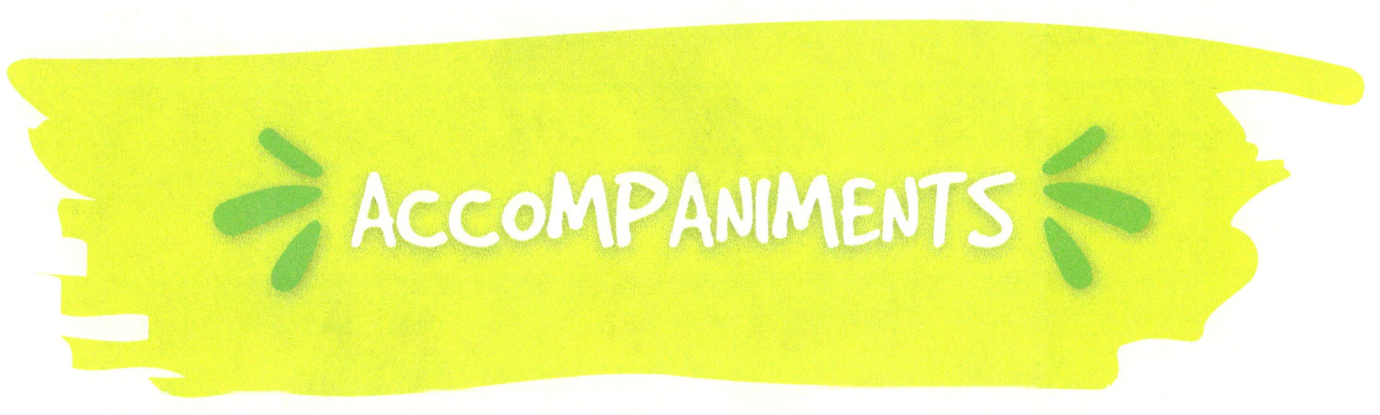

Homemade Vegan Butter

You will need:

125g almond flour

175ml unsweetened cashew hemp or almond milk

1/2 tsp Himalayan sea salt

1 tsp. apple cider vinegar

60ml avocado oil (or pure olive oil)

220ml melted raw coconut oil

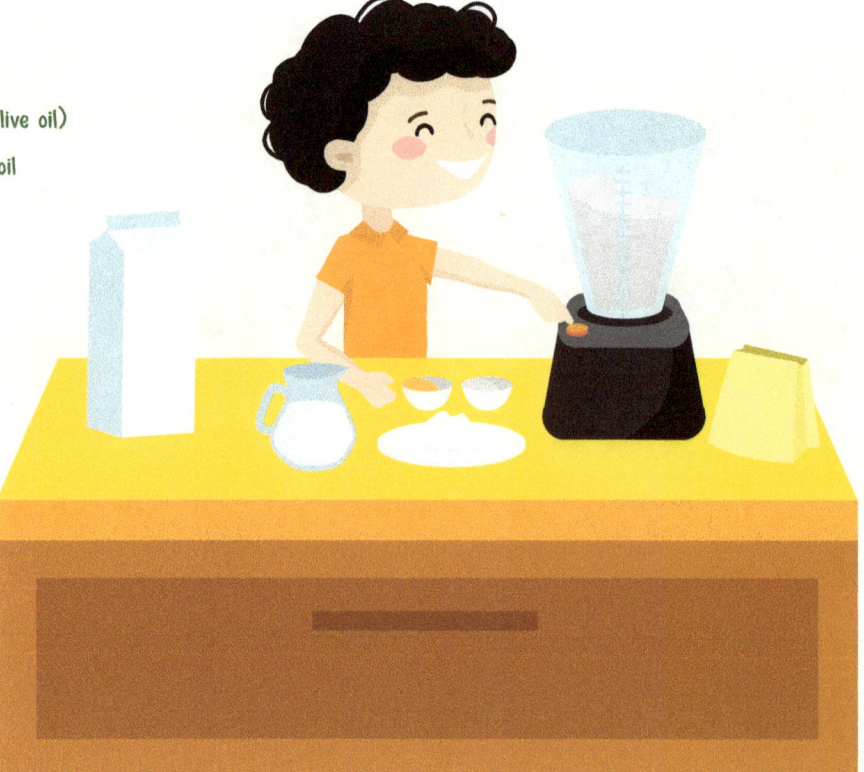

Page 142 MONSTER FIGHTING RECIPES

How to Make:

1. Mix the flour, milk and sea salt in the blender
2. Add the coconut and avocado oil and blend until completely smooth for at least 2 minutes – allow as much air to get in as possible
3. Pour into a container or silicone mould and place to fridge
4. This will take several hours to set and can be used as normal butter would be (use within 10-14 days)

TIP add some of the mix to an ice cube tray and freeze to last longer and for great use when cooking.

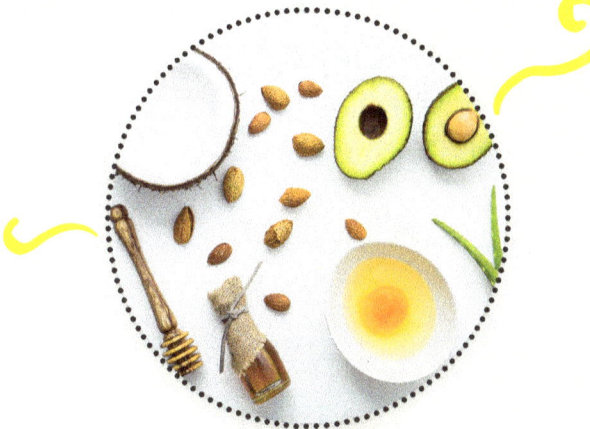

NUTRITIONAL VALUE:

Great source of Vitamins A, C, B1, B6, B9, B12, E, Iron, Magnesium, Calcium and Phosphorus, and a very good source of Fibre, Potassium, Copper and Manganese. Its nutrients and antioxidants may help to boost your immune system, protect your eyesight, lower your risk of certain cancers and promote heart and skin health. With ingredients that act as a natural antibacterial, antiseptic and antibiotic agent, full of anti-oxidants, anti-inflammatory and pain relieving properties, anti-fungal, anti-diabetic, analgesic, antipyretic, anticancer, and anti-tumorigenic properties, this recipe is powerful and healing.

South American Dressing

MAKES 200 ML

Ingredients:

Chopped coriander leaves 30 g (1/3 cup) (about 1 bunch)

Lime juice 125 ml (1/2 cup)

Extra-virgin olive oil 125 ml (1/2 cup)

Sea salt and freshly ground black pepper

Method:

1. Place the coriander, lime juice and olive oil in a bowl and mix to combine. Season with salt and pepper. Store in an airtight jar in the fridge for up to 1 week.

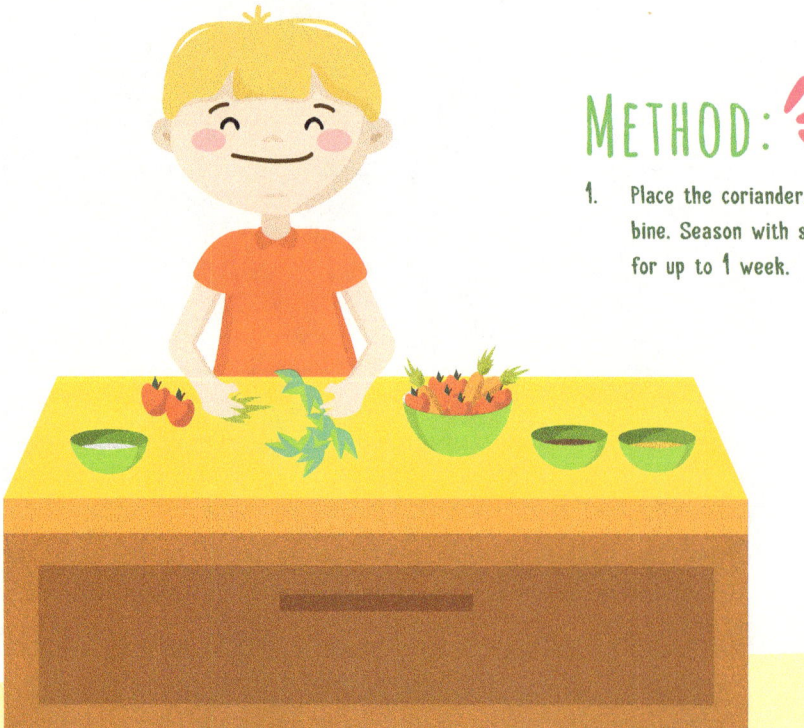

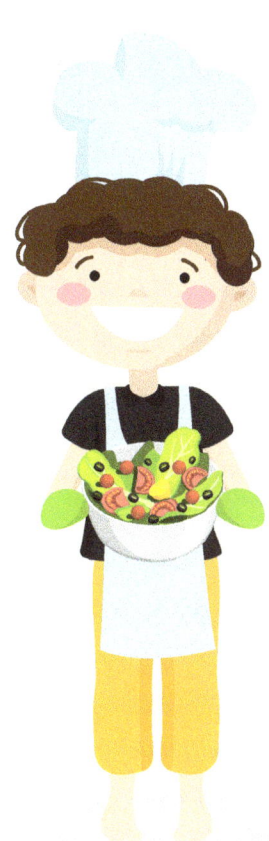

Note:

I use either coconut oil or good-quality animal fats for cooking as they have high smoke points (meaning they do not oxidise at high temperatures). Some of my favourite animal fats to use are lard (pork fat), tallow (rendered beef fat), rendered chicken fat and duck fat. These may be hard to find – ask at your local butcher or meat supplier, look online for meat suppliers who sell them or make your own when making bone broths.

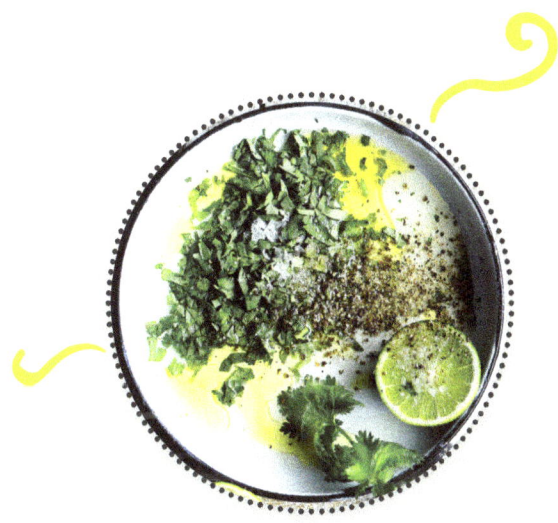